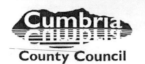

Good Me Bad Me

Good Me Bad Me

ALI LAND

MICHAEL JOSEPH
an imprint of
PENGUIN BOOKS

MICHAEL JOSEPH

UK | USA | Canada | Ireland | Australia
India | New Zealand | South Africa

Michael Joseph is part of the Penguin Random House group of companies
whose addresses can be found at global.penguinrandomhouse.com.

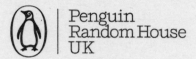

First published 2017
005

Copyright © Bo Dreams Ltd, 2017

The moral right of the author has been asserted

Set in 13/16.25 pt Bembo Book MT Std
Typeset by Jouve (UK), Milton Keynes
Printed in Great Britain by Clays Ltd, St Ives plc

A CIP catalogue record for this book is available from the British Library

HARDBACK ISBN: 978–0–718–18292–2
TRADE PAPERBACK ISBN: 978–0–718–18293–9

www.greenpenguin.co.uk

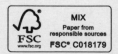

To mental health nurses everywhere. The true rock stars.
This book is for you.

'But the hearts of small children are delicate organs.
A cruel beginning in this world can twist them into
curious shapes.'

Carson McCullers, 1917–1967

Have you ever dreamt of a place far, far away? I have.

A field full of poppies.

Tiny red dancers, waltzing in glee.

Pointing their petals to a path that leads to a shoreline, clean. Unbroken.

Floating on my back, a turquoise ocean. Blue sky.

Nothing. Nobody.

I long to hear the words: 'I'll never let anything happen to you.' Or: 'It wasn't her fault, she was only a child.'

Yes, these are the kinds of dreams I have.

I don't know what's going to happen to me. I'm scared. Different. I wasn't given a choice.

I promise this.

I promise to be the best I can be.

I promise to try.

Up eight. Up another four.
The door on the right.

The playground.
That's what she called it.
Where the games were evil, and there was only ever one winner.
When it wasn't my turn, she made me watch.
A peephole in the wall.
Asked me afterwards. What did you see, Annie?
What did you see?

Forgive me when I tell you it was me.

It was me that told.

The detective. A kindly man, belly full and round. Disbelief at first. Then, the stained dungarees I pulled from my bag. Tiny.

The teddy bear on the front peppered red with blood. I could have brought more, so many to choose from. She never knew I kept them.

Shifted in his chair he did. Sat up straight, him and his gut.

His hand – I noticed a slight tremor as it reached for the telephone. Come now, he said. You need to hear this. The silent waiting for his superior to arrive. Bearable for me. Less so for him. A hundred questions beat a drum in his head. Is she telling the truth? Can't be. That many? Dead? Surely not.

I told the story again. And again. Same story. Different faces watched, different ears listened. I told them everything.

Well.

Almost everything.

The video recorder on, a gentle whirring the only noise in the room once I finished my statement.

You might have to go to court, you know that, right? You're the only witness, one of the detectives said. Another asked, do you think it's safe for us to send her home? If what she's saying is true? The chief inspector in charge replied, we'll have a team assembled in a matter of hours, then turned to me and said, nothing's going to happen to you. It already has, I wanted to reply.

Everything moved quickly after that, it had to. I was dropped off at the school gates, in an unmarked car, in time for pick-up. In time for her to pick me up. She would be waiting with her demands, recently more urgent than usual. Two in the last six months. Two little boys. Gone.

Act normal, they said. Go home. We're coming for her. Tonight.

The slow grind of the clock above my wardrobe. *Tick. Tock. Tick.* And they did. They came. The middle of the night, the element of surprise in their favour. A nearly imperceptible crunching on the gravel outside, I was downstairs by the time they forced their way through the door.

Shouting. A tall, thin man dressed in plain clothes, unlike the others. A string of commands sliced through the sour air of our living room. You, take upstairs. You, in there. You two take the cellar. You. You. You.

A tidal wave of blue uniforms scattered throughout our house. Guns held in praying hands, flat against their chests. The thrill of the search, along with the terror of the truth, etched in equal measure on their faces.

And then you.

Dragged from your room. A red crease of sleep visible down your cheek, eyes foggy with the adjustment from a state of rest to a state of arrest. You said nothing. Even when your face was mashed into the carpet, your rights read out, their knees and elbows pressed in your back. Your nightie rode high up your thighs. No underwear. The indignity of it all.

You turned your head to the side. Faced me. Your eyes never left mine, I read them with ease. You said nothing to them, yet everything to me. I nodded.

But only when no one was watching.

2

New name. New family.
Shiny.
New.
Me.

My foster dad Mike's a psychologist, an expert in trauma; so is his daughter, Phoebe, although more in the causing than the healing. Saskia, the mother. I think she's trying to make me feel at home, although I'm not sure, she's very different from you, Mummy. Skinny and vacant.

Lucky, the staff at the unit told me while I waited for Mike to come. What a fantastic family the Newmonts are, and a place at Wetherbridge. Wow. Wow. WOW. Yes, I get it. I should feel lucky, but really I'm scared. Scared of finding out who and what I might be.

Scared of them finding out, too.

A week ago now Mike came to collect me, towards the end of the summer holidays. My hair brushed neat, pulled back in a band, I practised how to speak, should I sit or stand. Every minute that went by, when the voices I heard weren't his, the nurses instead, sharing a joke, I became convinced he and his family had changed their minds. Come to their senses. I stood rooted to the spot, waiting to be told, sorry, you won't be going anywhere today.

But then he arrived. Greeted me with a smile, a firm handshake, not formal, but nice, nice to know he wasn't afraid to connect. To run the risk of being contaminated. I remember him noticing my lack of belongings, one small suitcase. In it, a few books, some clothes and other things hidden too, memories of you. Of us. The rest, taken as evidence when our house was stripped bare. Not to worry, he said, we'll organize a shopping trip. Saskia and Phoebe are at home, he added, we'll all have dinner together, a real welcome.

We met with the head of the unit. Gently, gently, he said, take each day as it comes. I wanted to tell him, it's the nights I fear.

Smiles exchanged. Handshakes. Mike signed on the line, turned to face me and said, ready?

Not really, no.

But I left with him anyway.

The drive home was short, less than an hour. Every street and building new to me. It was light when we got there, a big house, white pillars at the front. Okay? asked Mike. I nodded, though I didn't feel okay. I waited for him to unlock the front door; my heart spiralled up into my throat when I realized it wasn't locked. We walked straight in, could have been anyone. He called out to his wife, I'd met her a few times now. Sas, he said, we're home. Coming, was the reply. Hi, Milly, she said, welcome. I smiled, that's what I thought I should do. Rosie, their terrier, greeted me too, jumped at my legs, sneezed with joy when I reached for her ears, gave them a rub. Where's Phoebs? Mike asked. On her way back from Clondine's, Saskia replied. Perfect, he said, dinner in half an hour or so then. He suggested Saskia should show me to my room, I remember him nodding at her in a way that looked like encouragement. For her, not me.

8

I followed her up the stairs, tried not to count. New home. New me.

It's just you and Phoebe on the third floor, Saskia explained, we're on the next level down. We've given you the room at the back, it has a nice view of the garden from the balcony.

It was the yellow of the sunflowers I saw first. Brightly coloured. Smiles in a vase. I thanked her, told her they were one of my favourite flowers, she looked pleased. Feel free to explore, she said, there's some clothes in the wardrobe, we'll get you more of course, you can choose them. She asked me if I needed anything, no, I replied, and she left.

I put my suitcase down, walked over to the balcony door, checked it was locked. Secure. The wardrobe to the right, tall, antique pine. I didn't look inside, I didn't want to think about putting on clothes, taking them off. As I turned round, I noticed drawers under the bed, opened them, ran my hands along the back and the sides – nothing there. Safe, for now. An en suite, large, the entire wall on the right covered with a mirror. I turned away from my reflection, didn't want to be reminded. I checked the lock on the bathroom door worked, and that it couldn't be opened from the outside, then I sat on the bed and tried not to think about you.

Before long, I heard feet pounding up the stairs. I tried to stay calm, to remember the breathing exercises I'd been shown by my psychologist, but my head felt fuzzy, so when she appeared at my door I focused on her forehead, as close to eye contact as I could manage. Dinner's ready, her voice more like a purr, creamy, a dash of snide, just as I remembered her from when we met with the social worker. We couldn't meet at the unit, she wasn't allowed to know the truth, or be given the opportunity to wonder. I remember feeling intimidated. The way she looked, blonde and self-assured, bored, forced to welcome strangers into her home. Twice during the meeting she asked how long I'd be staying. Twice she was shushed.

Dad asked me to come and get you, she said, her arms folded across her chest. Defensive. I'd seen the staff at the unit calling patients out on what their body language meant, labelling it. I quietly watched, learnt a lot. It's days ago now, but the last thing she said before she turned on her heels like an angry ballerina stuck in my head: Oh, and welcome to the mad house.

I followed her smell, sweet and pink, down to the kitchen, fantasizing about what having a sister might be like. What sort of sisters she and I might become. She would be Meg, I thought, I would be Jo, little women of our own. I'd been told at the unit, hope was my best weapon, it would be what got me through.

Foolishly, I believed them.

3

I slept in my clothes that first night. Silk pyjamas chosen by Saskia remained unworn, touched only to move them from my bed. The material slippery on my skin. I'm able to sleep better now, if only for part of the night. I've come a long way since I left you. The staff at the unit told me I didn't speak for the first three days. I sat on the bed, back against the wall. Stared. Silent. Shock they called it. Something much worse, I wanted to say. Something that came into my room every time I allowed myself to sleep. Moved in a slither, under the door, hissed at me, called itself Mummy. Still does.

When I can't sleep, it's not sheep I count, it's days until the trial. Me against you. Everybody against you. Twelve weeks on Monday. Eighty-eight days, and counting. I count up, I count down. I count until I cry, and again until I stop, and I know it's wrong but, somewhere in the numbers, I begin to miss you. I'm going to have to work hard between now and then. There are things I must put right in my head. Things I must get right if I'm called upon to present in court. So much can go wrong when all eyes are looking the same way.

Mike has a big part to play in the work to be done. A treatment plan drawn up between him and the unit staff detailed a weekly therapy session with me in the run-up to the trial. An opportunity for me to discuss any concerns or worries with him. Yesterday he suggested Wednesdays, midway through each week. I said yes, not because I wanted to. But because he wanted me to, he thinks it will help.

School begins tomorrow, we're all in the kitchen. Phoebe's saying thank god, can't wait to get back, and out of this house. Mike laughs it off, Saskia looks sad. Over the past week I've noticed something's not right between her and Phoebe. They exist almost entirely independently of each other, Mike the translator, the mediator. Sometimes Phoebe calls her Saskia, not Mum. I expected her to be punished the first time I heard her say it, but no. Not that I've seen. I also haven't seen them touch each other, and I think touch is an indicator of love. Not the kind of touch you experienced though, Milly. There is good touch and bad touch, said the staff at the unit.

Phoebe announces she's going out to meet someone called Izzy, who just got back from France. Mike suggests she take me too, introduce me. She rolls her eyes and says come on, I haven't seen Iz all summer, she can meet her tomorrow. It'll be nice for Milly to meet one of the girls, he persists, take her to some of the places you hang out. Fine, she agrees, but it's not really my job.

'It's nice of you though,' says Saskia.

She stares her mother down. Stares and stares, until she wins. Saskia looks away, a pink flush imprinting on her cheeks.

'I was just saying how nice I thought you were being.'

'Yeah, well, nobody asked you, did they?'

I wait for the backlash, a hand or an object. But nothing. Only Mike.

'Please don't speak to your mother like that.'

When we leave the house there's a girl in a tracksuit

sitting on the wall opposite our driveway, she looks at us as we pass. Phoebe says fuck off you little shit, find another wall to sit on. The girl responds by giving her the finger.

'Who was that?' I ask.

'Just some skanky kid from the estate.'

She nods towards the tower blocks on the left-hand side of our road.

'Don't get used to this by the way, I'll be doing my own thing when school kicks off properly.'

'Okay.'

'The close just there runs right past our garden, there's nothing much up there, a few garages and stuff, and it's quicker to get to school this way.'

'What time do you normally leave in the morning?'

'It depends. I usually meet Iz and we walk together. Sometimes we go to Starbucks and hang out for a bit, but it's hockey season this term and I'm captain so I'll be leaving early most mornings doing fitness and stuff.'

'You must be really good if you're captain.'

'Suppose so. So what's your story then? Where are your folks?'

An invisible hand reaches into the pit of my stomach, squeezes it hard, doesn't let go. I feel my head fill up again. Relax, I tell myself, I practised these questions with the staff at the unit, over and over again.

'My mum left when I was young, I lived with my dad but he died recently.'

'Fuck, that's pretty shit.'

I nod, leave it at that. Less is more, I was told.

'Dad probably showed you some of this stuff last week but at the end of our road, just here, there's a short-cut to school that way.'

She points to the right.

'Cross over the road, take the first left and then the second street on the right, it takes about five minutes from there.'

I'm about to thank her but she's distracted, her face breaking into a smile. I follow her gaze and see a blonde girl crossing the road towards us, blowing exaggerated air kisses. Phoebe laughs and waves, says, that's Iz. Her legs glow brown against the ripped denim shorts she's wearing, and like Phoebe, she's pretty. Very pretty. I watch the way they greet each other, drape round each other, a conversation begins a hundred miles an hour. Questions are flung, returned, they pull their phones out of their pockets, compare photos. They snigger about boys, and a girl named Jacinta who Izzy says is an absolute fright in her bikini, I swear the whole fucking pool emptied when she went for a swim. This whole interaction takes only minutes, but with the awkwardness of being ignored, it feels like hours. It's Izzy who looks at me, then says to Phoebe, 'Who's this then, the newest newbie at Mike's rescue centre?'

Phoebe laughs and replies, 'She's called Milly. She's staying with us for a bit.'

'Thought your dad wasn't taking anyone else in?'

'Whatever. You know he can't help himself when it comes to strays.'

'Are you coming to Wetherbridge?' Izzy asks me.

'Yes.'

'Are you from London?'

'No.'

'Do you have a boyfriend?'

'No.'

'Crikey, do you only speak in robot tongue? Yes. No.

14

No.' She waves her arms around, makes a mechanical noise like the Dalek from the *Doctor Who* episode I watched in a drama lesson at my old school. They both erupt into laughter, return to their phones. I wish I could tell them I speak like that, slow and purposeful, when I'm nervous and to filter the noise. White noise, punctuated by your voice. Even now, especially now, you're here, in my head. Normal behaviour required little effort for you, but for me, an avalanche. I was always surprised by how much they loved you at your work. No violence or rage, your smile gentle, your voice soothing. In the palm of your hand you kept them, isolated them. Took the women you knew could be persuaded to one side, talked close in their ears. Secure. Loved. That's how you made them feel, that's why they trusted you with their children.

'I might head home, I'm not feeling so good.'

'Fine,' Phoebe replies. 'Just don't get me in trouble with Dad.'

Izzy looks up, a provocative smile. 'See you at school,' she says, and as I walk away I hear her add: 'This should be fun.'

The girl in the tracksuit is no longer on the wall. I pause to look into the estate, follow the tower blocks up to the sky, my neck craning backwards. There were no tower blocks in Devon, just houses and fields. Acres of privacy.

When I go back into the house, Mike asks me where Phoebe is. I explain about Izzy, he smiles, an apology I think.

'They've been friends for ever,' he says. 'A whole summer to catch up on. Do you fancy a quick chat in my study, touch base before school tomorrow?'

I say yes — I seem to be saying it a lot, it's a good word,

one I can hide behind. Mike's study is large with bay windows overlooking the garden. A mahogany-coloured desk, a photo frame and a green antique-style reading lamp, piles of paper. There's a home library, rows of built-in shelves full of books, the remaining walls painted a mauve colour. It feels stable. Safe. He sees me looking at the shelves, laughs. I know, I know, he says, far too many, but between you and me, I don't think you can ever have too many books.

I nod, agree.

'Did you have a good library at your school?' he asks.

I don't like the question. I don't like thinking about life, the way it was before. But I answer, show willing.

'Not really, but there was one in the village next to ours, I went there sometimes.'

'Reading's very therapeutic, just let me know if you'd like to borrow anything. I've plenty, as you can see.'

He winks, but not in a way that makes me feel uncomfortable, gestures to an armchair, take a seat. Relax. I sit down, notice the door to the study is closed, Mike must have done it when I was looking at his books. He refers to the chair I'm sitting in.

'It's comfy, isn't it?' he says.

I nod, try to look more relaxed, more comfy. I want to get it right. It also reclines, he adds, you just need to flick the lever on the side, if it takes your fancy, go for it. It doesn't, and I don't. The thought of being alone with someone in a room on a chair that reclines, me on my back. No. I don't like that idea.

'I know we discussed this at the unit before you were discharged but it's important to go over what we agreed before the next few weeks of school swallow you up.'

One of my feet begins to jiggle. He looks down at it.

'You look unsure.'

'A little bit.'

'All I ask is that you keep an open mind, Milly. View these sessions as moments of respite, somewhere to pause and take a breath. We've got just under three months until the court case starts so partly we'll be working on preparing you for that, but we'll also continue with the guided relaxation the unit psychologist started with you.'

'Do we still have to do that?'

'Yes, it'll be helpful for you in the long run.'

How can I tell him it won't, not if things that frighten me find a way out.

'It's human nature to want to avoid the things we feel threatened by, Milly, the things that make us feel less in control, but it's important we go there. Begin the process of putting things to rest. I'd like you to think of a place that feels safe for you, I'm going to ask you to tell me about it next time we meet. Initially it might feel like a difficult thing to do, but I need you to try. It can be anywhere, a classroom at your old school, a bus journey you used to take.'

She drove me to school. Every day.

'Or somewhere in the village you lived next to, like a cafe or the library you mentioned, anywhere as long as the feeling you associate with it is a comforting one. Does that make sense?'

'I'll try.'

'Good. Now, what about tomorrow, how are you feeling? It's never easy being the new girl.'

'I'm looking forward to being busy, it helps.'

'Well, just make sure and ease yourself in, it can be quite

full-on at Wetherbridge but I've no doubt you'll keep up. Is there anything else you'd like to talk about or ask, anything you're feeling unsure about?'

Everything.

'No, thank you.'

'Let's leave it at that for tonight then but if anything does crop up in between now and our first session, my door's always open.'

As I go back to my room I can't help but feel frustrated that Mike wants to continue with the hypnosis. He thinks by calling it 'guided relaxation' I won't recognize it for what it is, but I do. I overheard the psychologist at the unit telling a colleague that the hypnosis technique he'd been using on me would hopefully be a good way to *unlock* me. Better left locked, I wanted to tell him.

I hear music as I pass Phoebe's room so she must be back. I work up the courage to knock on her door, I want to ask her what to expect at school tomorrow.

'Who is it?' she shouts.

'Milly,' I reply.

'I'm busy getting ready for tomorrow,' she responds, 'you should do the same.'

I whisper my reply through the wood – *I'm scared* – then I go into my room, lay out my new uniform. A blue skirt, white shirt and a stripy tie, two shades of blue. And try as I might not to think of you, it's all I can do. Our daily drive to and from school, you worked the early shift so I wouldn't have to get the bus. An opportunity to remind me, the song you sang as you pinched me. How my mouth watered with pain. Our secrets are special, you'd say, when the chorus came on, they're between me and you.

Just after nine p.m. Saskia comes in to say goodnight.

Try not to worry about tomorrow, she says, Wetherbridge is a really lovely school. After she closes my door I hear her at Phoebe's. She knocks, then opens it. I hear Phoebe respond — What do you want?

Just checking you're all set for the morning. Whatever, Phoebe replies, and the door closes again.

4

I made it through the first two days of school, Thursday and Friday last week, without incident, sheltered by the induction programme. Lectures on rules and expectations, an introduction to my guidance teacher, Miss Kemp. Year Elevens don't normally get guidance teachers but as I'm the only new arrival in the year, and she teaches art, I was paired with her. The headmistress from my old school sent a letter via social services, explained the talent she thought I had for art. Miss Kemp seemed excited, said she couldn't wait to see what I could do. She came across as nice, kind, although you can never tell. Not really. I remember her smell more than anything, tobacco mixed with something else I couldn't put my finger on. Familiar though.

The weekend was quiet. Mike works Saturdays at his practice in Notting Hill Gate – where the real money comes from. Saskia was in and out of the house, yoga and other things. Phoebe at Izzy's. A lot of 'me' time. On Sunday evening Mike and Saskia took me to a cinema called the Electric on Portobello Road, and even though it was so different from those movie nights we used to have at home, I spent the entire time thinking about you.

When we got back, Phoebe was in the games room, wandered out looking angry. How cosy, she said. We asked you if you wanted to come, Mike replied. She shrugged, yeah, well, I wasn't back from Iz's in time, was I?

She and I walked upstairs together. Looks like you're settling in nicely, doesn't it, she said to me. Enjoy it while it lasts, you won't be here that long, no one ever is. I felt it, deep in my gut. An alarm. A signal.

The next morning at breakfast it's only Mike and me. He explains Saskia's having a lie-in, catching up on some sleep. He doesn't know that I've seen the pills in her handbag.

Unfortunately Phoebe's gone already, he says. Would you like me to walk with you, it's your first full week? I tell him I'll be fine on my own though I'm not sure it's true. During my two days of induction I had lunch with the other girls in the canteen. Curiosity at first, soon became disinterest when word spread — she speaks like a robot, stares at her feet. Freak. I hid the fact my hands sometimes shake — permanent damage to my nervous system — by putting them in my blazer pocket, or carrying a folder. It's clear things move fast at this school, ruled in or out in the blink of an eye. No point looking to Phoebe, it's obvious she prefers not to associate with me, so I'm ignored, firmly in the category of outsider. THE outsider.

But today, Monday, is different.

Today, a wave of nudges and sniggers from the girls in my year ripple with intent as I cross the school courtyard.

I'm noticed.

I take a hard right once inside, keen to avoid the middle corridor, a gauntlet, a gathering place of catty, snobby, beautiful girls. I leave behind the sniggers I can hear, the high-pitched insults traded so easily between them, even the ones that are friends — especially the ones that are friends — and head to the locker room.

I use my back to open the door. Arms full of folders.

I turn. See it immediately.

SUPERSIZED. Taped to the front of my locker. My school photo, taken last week on my first day. Awkward and unsure. Ugly. Mouth slightly open, enough to be stuffed with an image of an oversized penis, a speech bubble.

MILLY FUCKS WILLY

I move, let the door close. A gentle shunt seals the room. I'm drawn towards the poster. Towards me. Curious to see me in a way I have never. A pink, veiny intruder juts out of my mouth. I tilt my head, picture myself biting down. Hard.

A blast of noise bleeds in from the corridor as the door opens and closes again. The soft steps of the person behind me. I pull the poster down at the same time as a hand reaches out, rests on my shoulder. The clunking of her heavy bracelets; her distinctive aroma wraps round me like a blanket on a day already too warm. I curse myself for pausing. She saw it before I pulled it down, I know she did. Idiot. I should know better. You taught me better than that.

'What's that in your hand, Milly?'

'Nothing, Miss Kemp, it's fine.'

Leave me alone.

'Come on now, you can tell me.'

'There's nothing to tell.'

The bulky assortment of her rings. I feel them against my collarbone as she guides me round to face her. Invested already, I can sense it, and if what I've overheard in conversations between the girls – about her being a bit silly, a bit

23

over-involved at times – is true, I know she won't let this drop. My eyes, trained on the ground, move to her feet. Chunky hippy clogs, heavy wooden soles. The longer I stare, the more they look like two boats marooned ashore, stuck in a secret sandbank under her skirt. *Sail away, leave me alone.*

'It doesn't look like nothing, let me see.'

I crumple it into the small of my back. Pray a silent spell. Make me vanish, or her. Good. Better.

'I'll be late, I should go.'

'I'm not letting you leave feeling like this. Show me, I might be able to help.'

Her voice, the way she uses it, musical almost. I feel better, a bit. My eyes travel up. Shins. She's new to me. Be cautious, yes, my psychologist said, but remember most people are not a threat. Thighs. More hippy shit, dippy shit. A corduroy skirt, a paisley shirt, a walking project not quite finished, the kind of chaotic style you'd hate, Mummy. Colours and layers. Layers and colours. Hands twist round each other, oversized rings clink and collide, dodgem cars. Nervous? No. Something else. Anticipation. Yes. A moment between us. A bonding, she thinks. Her smell, less oppressive now. I make it to her eyes. Hazel and flicky, dark and light, her hand stretches out towards me.

'Let me see.'

The bell goes so I hand her the poster, I don't want to be late for class, another reason to be singled out. She attempts to smooth out the creases in the paper, flattens it on to her thigh, rubs it with her hand, an ironing motion. I look away. I hear her breath deepen as if trying to hold something in. How could they? she says. Reaches out to me, her hand on my blazer sleeve, not my skin. Thankfully.

'I'd rather forget about it, Miss.'

'No, I'm afraid not, I'll have to get to the bottom of this, especially as I'm your guidance teacher. Do you have any idea who's behind it?'

I reply no, though it's not strictly true. Last week, on the street.

Izzy's words: This should be fun.

'I'll be making sure I find out, Milly, don't you worry.'

I want to tell her not to bother, there's been worse, but I can't – she doesn't know who I am, where I've come from. As she looks down at the poster again my eyes are drawn to her neck. The pulse, strong and steady. Each time it beats, the surrounding skin quivers a little. The thought is shaken from my head when Phoebe and Izzy crash through the door, stopping short when they realize I have company. It's clear they came to gloat, phones poised in their hands. Capture the moment. The edgy glances back and forth between the two of them, evidence enough. I never get why people aren't better at hiding how they feel, although it's fair to say I've had more practice than most. Miss Kemp clocks them looking at each other, comes to her own conclusion. The right one. Maybe she's not as daft or silly as the girls think.

'Surely not? And Phoebe, especially you, how could you? What would your parents say about this? They'd be furious. I don't know, I just don't know any more, you girls, the way you treat each other. I'll need to think about this, both of you report to me in the art room after registration and –'

'But, Miss Kemp, there's a meeting about the half-term hockey tour, I have to be there, I'm captain.'

'Please do not interrupt me, Phoebe, understood? You

and Izzy will be in my classroom by eight fifty-five at the latest otherwise this matter will go further, much further. Got it?'

A silence, no longer than a few seconds. Izzy speaks.

'Yes, Miss Kemp.'

'Good, now go and sign in, then straight to my room. Milly, you'd also better sign in, and don't worry, I'll sort this.'

My heart hammers all the way to registration. Miss Kemp, too busy being 'involved', failed to see the gesture Phoebe gave me as we left the lockers. A single finger across her throat. Eyes fixed on me. Dead meat. Me. Dead meat.

As if.

Phoebe, darling.

5

Less than two hours later, outside the tuck shop, they approach from either side, press against me. A glossy, hair-flicking version of the game sardines.

'How's life as Miss Kemp's new little bitch?' Izzy's hot breath in my left ear.

Phoebe, nowhere to be seen. She's smarter than that. Step forward Clondine, her other best friend, keen to please, on my right, sleeves firmly rolled up. The toilets behind the science block, hardly ever used, spell trouble. Hands push me through the door. Push, shove, a final push.

They waste no time.

'You think you're so clever, don't you? Telling your little Miss Kemp on us.'

'I didn't tell her.'

'Do you hear that, Clondine, she's denying it.'

'Oh, I hear her all right, I just don't fucking believe her.'

Izzy moves in, phone in one hand. Films us. Shoves me. Hard. A smell of strawberries on her breath, so enticing I could crawl into her mouth. Bubblegum visible through her clicky-clacky cheerleader teeth, no braces like Clondine, a mouthful of coloured metal. She rests her hand on the wall above my head, wants me to feel small. Threatened. A scene from a movie she watched. She blows a bubble. Pink and opaque. It connects with my nose, collapses over it. Giggles erupt. Izzy backs away, Clondine picks up where she left off.

'Give me your number, and don't say you haven't got a phone, Phoebe told us Mike bought you one.'

Silence.

Your voice in my head. THAT'S MY GIRL, YOU SHOW THEM. THANKFUL NOW, YOU SHOULD BE, FOR THE LESSONS I TAUGHT YOU, ANNIE. Your praise, so rare, when it comes, rips through me like a bush fire swallowing houses and trees, and other teenage girls who are less strong, in its hot hungry mouth. I meet their stares, the remnants of Izzy's gum hanging off my chin. Thrown by my defiance, they are, I see it. Fleeting. The twitch around their succulent lips, eyes slightly wider. I shake my head, slow and deliberate. Izzy, the hungrier of the two, takes the bait.

'Give me your goddamn phone number, bitch.'

Her hands push me, her face presses against mine, I welcome the contact. I am real. See me, feel me, but know that I come from a place where this is merely a warm-up.

I shake my head again.

A stinging sensation sweeps across my cheek, into my ear, out the other side. Slapped. I hear laughter, admiration at Izzy's performance. My eyes are closed but I imagine her taking a bow, ever the crowd-pleaser. Her voice is faint, the ringing in my ear threatens to drown it out, but the words are unmistakable.

'I. Won't. Ask. Again.'

And I never forget.

Never.

When they get what they want, they leave. My hand touches the heat on my cheek and I'm reminded of you. Swallowed. A vortex of memories. We're back in our house, I can smell the lavender you loved, the vase in the bathroom. It's the night of your arrest, I'd been at the police station all afternoon. I faked a letter from you, gave it to the school office, I was excused after lunch, no questions asked.

I was terrified to look at you that night, to meet your eyes, as if the secret shame of what I'd done was scrawled. Spray-painted, on my face. I offered to do the ironing, anything to stop my hands from shaking, and so I'd be armed if the police came early and you went for me. You looked different, smaller, still intimidating but less so. But it wasn't you who'd changed, it was me. The end in sight. Or the beginning.

I worried they might not come, change their minds, decide I was making it up. I tried to breathe normally, stand normally, not that it mattered since you could flip at any given moment. One minute you'd be arranging flowers, the next you'd demand I put on a show. There aren't many everyday activities left that don't remind me of you, of how you liked to do them. When bedtime came I waited to be told where I was to sleep. Sometimes in your bed, other times I'd be given a reprieve and sent to mine. The funny thing, or sad, was part of me wanted to sleep with you that night knowing it would be our last, and another part of me was too scared to go upstairs on my own. Up eight, up another four, the door on the right. Opposite mine. The playground.

You said nothing as you closed your bedroom door, it was one of those nights. You could go days without talking to or acknowledging me then swallow me up, my skin, my hair, in minutes, anything you could grab. I said goodbye that night, whispered it. I think I might have also said, I love you, and I did. Still do, though I'm trying not to.

When I went upstairs I leant into the corridor wall

outside the room opposite mine, needed to feel something solid against me, yet I soon moved. I heard them. The voices of tiny ghosts bleeding out of the wall. Swooping. Plummeting. A no man's land.

She'll be there, waiting, the girl who gave Phoebe the finger, I know she will. I've seen her a couple of times since that first night. I turn the corner into my road, there she is, sitting on the wall. I feel something in my tummy, a squeeze, not fear. Pleasure, I think. Excitement. She's small, alone. I haven't spoken to her yet but I'm working on it. As I walk closer she begins to swing her legs up and down, hits the bricks of the wall that surrounds her estate opposite my house with alternating thumps. Her right eye, bruised and swollen, only open a little. A football strip, all blue. Her open eye stares at me as I walk past. It blinks, blinks again. A one-eyed Morse code. I pull the crisps out, the bag opens with a pop, it knows it has a part to play. I glance at her. Her good eye looks away, a chirpy whistle starts up, she's all freckles and aloof. I shrug, cross the road. Three. Two . . .

'You got anything to eat?'

One.

I turn to face her – 'You can have some of my crisps if you like?'

She looks around, over her shoulder, as if checking we're alone, then asks, 'What flavour are they?'

'Salt and vinegar.'

I walk towards her, hold the packet out. If she wants them she'll have to leave the wall. She does. Quick as a flash, takes them, sits back down. Her scuffed trainers resume their dance: *thump, thump,* right, left. I ask her name but she ignores me. It takes only minutes, she shovels, more than eats the crisps. Devours them. Tips up the packet so it covers her mouth, taps it on the bottom, the remaining crumbs, gone. The empty bag floats to the ground. She's older than she looks, twelve or thirteen maybe. Small for her age.

'You got anything else?'

'No, nothing.'

She blows a saliva bubble which is both disgusting and fascinating. The way it forms on her lips, the way she sucks it back in. Bold, yet babyish, all at once. I want to ask her why she sits here so often on her own, why a wall on a street is better than home, but she leaves. Swivels her legs over the back of the wall, walks away, towards one of the tower blocks. I watch her go, she knows somehow, feels my stare. Turns round, gives me a look that I think says, what's your problem. I smile in response, she shrugs over her shoulder at me. I try again.

'What's your name?' I call out.

She stops walking, turns her body round to face me, scuffs one of her trainers into the ground. Once. Twice.

'Who wants to know?'

'Milly, my name's Milly.'

She scrunches her eyes, a flash of uncertainty across her face, but answers anyway.

'Morgan,' she says.

'That's a nice name.'

'Whatever,' she replies, peels into a jog and is soon out of sight. As I cross the road I roll the letters of her name up and in, over my tongue and lips, and while I search for the keys in my bag I can't help but feel pleased. I stood up for myself with Clondine and Izzy, and spoke to the girl on the wall. I can do this, I can do life after you.

31

6

I've managed to keep your night-time visits a secret so far.

The fact you come as a snake, underneath the door. Up into my bed. Lie your scaly body next to mine, measure me. Remind me I still belong to you. I end up on the floor by morning, curled in a ball, the duvet over my head. My skin is hot, yet inside I'm cold, it's hard to explain. I read in a book once that people who are violent are hot-headed, while psychopaths are cold-hearted. Hot and cold. Head and heart. But what if you come from a person who's both? What happens then?

Tomorrow, Mike and I are due to meet the prosecution lawyers. The men or women recruited to take you down. Throw away the key. Do you sit in your cell and wonder why? Why I left when I did when so many years had already gone by? There are two reasons but only one I can talk about, and it's this.

Sweet sixteen, mine. It's not until December though you began planning it months ago, but not in the way a mother should. A birthday you'll never forget, you said. Or survive, I remember thinking. Emails started to arrive from others you'd met. The dark belly of the internet. A shortlist. Three men and a woman, you invited them to come, share in the fun. Share me. It was to be my birthday, but I was the present. The piñata to punch. Sweet sixteen, you said, you couldn't wait. The words like sugary treats in your mouth. Lemons for me. Bitter and sour.

I feel the beginnings of a migraine as I get ready for school, another little gift left over from you. The buttons on my shirt defy my fingers, like trying to thread a needle with chopsticks. It takes me longer than usual, and by the time I pass Phoebe's room, the door's closed and I wonder if she's already left. I haven't seen her since yesterday in the locker room at school. I hope she and the girls have had enough 'fun' with me now.

Three flights up we are, thick cream carpet. Changes to tiles once you reach the hallway below. I misjudge the last step and trip, landing on the cold marble. I must have called out because Mike comes out of the kitchen.

'Easy now,' he says. 'Let me help you.'

He moves me on to the bottom step of the staircase, sits next to me. Stupid, I tell him. 'Not to worry,' he replies. 'Easily done, the house is still new to you. You're shading your eyes from the light, is it a migraine?'

'I think so.'

'We were told to expect these. It's probably best if you stay off school, certainly for the morning anyway. Try and sleep it off.'

My first instinct is no, but then I remember where I am – and where you are. Sometimes you'd take a Friday off work, a long weekend. You'd call school, tell them I was sick, a stomach bug or flu. Three whole days, just me and you.

'The kettle's boiled, I'll make you some tea then back to bed, okay?'

I nod, he helps me up. I ask him where Phoebe and Saskia are, they've gone already, he explains.

'Which reminds me, Sas left you a present in the kitchen.'

34

The present is small, shaped like a square. Wrapped in blue paper, a red bow.

'Open it if you like.'

The gesture is kind. I sit down at the table and as I watch Mike make the tea, the gentle way he lifts things, places them down, I'm flooded with gratitude. Not many people would take someone like me in, not many people would want that responsibility. That risk. I fight back the tears but they win. Land on the lilac tablecloth. Mike notices as he brings the mugs over, sits in the chair next to me. He looks at the unopened present in my hand, tells me not to worry. Take your time, he says, drink the tea, there's some honey in it, the sweetness will help.

He's right, and the warmth.

'I know it's only Tuesday but we should meet later, if you're up to it. I think you'd benefit from some time today, what do you think?'

I nod, though I want to say no. I don't want him to trample, wade through my inner thoughts and desires. He'd be disgusted to know I miss you, am missing you now as I sit here. When I opened the curtains this morning I noticed a bird box in the neighbours' garden and it reminded me of the time we built one together. You used a hammer to bang in the nails. When I asked to have a go, you stroked my hair, said yes, but be careful with your fingers. The nurse in you, thinking about preventing pain rather than causing it, for once.

'Good to see you've got some colour back. Why don't you head up to bed and I'll wake you later?'

I manage to sleep for the rest of the morning. Mike works from home for the day and we have lunch together, soup prepared for us by Sevita the housekeeper, and ham sandwiches. Rosie sits with her nose almost touching my leg, dewy brown eyes boring into my side. I slip her a piece of meat while we clear the table.

The lighting is kind in Mike's study, two lamps, nothing on overhead. He explains he'll drop the blinds but keep the shutters open. The blinds have elaborate purple pom-poms at the end of their ropes. He follows my gaze, smiles.

'Sas. She's the artistic one, not me.'

He walks to his desk, closes the lid of his laptop, takes his glasses off. Take a seat, he says, pointing to the armchair I sat in last time. I count as I sit, backwards from ten, try to calm my breathing. He picks up a cushion from one of the other armchairs. Blue velvet. Walks over to me, places it on the arm of the chair I'm sitting in. Smiles. He sits down opposite me, crosses his legs, interlocks his fingers, his elbows resting on the arms of the chair.

'I'm sure tomorrow's been on your mind, the meeting with June and the lawyers. You remember June, don't you? She's your Witness Case Officer, you met briefly in hospital.'

I nod.

'We'll be discussing a few things, but primarily the fact you might be cross-examined on your evidence.'

I reach for the cushion, hold it into my body.

'I know this is hard for you, Milly, and I know how painful it was giving a statement against your mother in the first place, but whatever happens we'll get you through it.'

'What will they want to ask? Will I have to tell them everything all over again?'

'We're not a hundred per cent sure yet, the prosecution

lawyers are working on finding out what the defence are up to.'

I wish I could tell him it's not the defence they need to worry about, it's you. The hours and hours spent every day, confined to a cell, you'll be putting them to good use. I know you will. You'll be thinking up a plan.

'You look troubled, Milly. What are you thinking about?'

That if I'd gone to the police sooner, Daniel, the last boy you took, would still be alive.

'Nothing really. I was just wondering if the lawyers that are defending my mum have been given a copy of my statement?'

'Yes, they have, and likely that's what you'll be questioned on. You're the key witness in your mother's trial and the defence will look to find ways to undermine your statement, try and create reasonable doubt around certain events.'

'What if I mess up, or I say the wrong thing?'

'I don't want you to worry about that at the moment. We've plenty of time to prepare if you are called upon. Hopefully we'll find out a bit more tomorrow. But what's important here is that you remember you're not the one on trial. Okay?'

I nod, say yes. For now, I think.

As soon as Mike starts I realize he's better than the unit psychologist, or maybe I'm just more comfortable with him. I want to move on from the past. I do. Yet even so, I try to resist relaxing into the session. My hands clench into fists, he tells me to unclench, concentrate on breathing. Close your eyes, rest your head on the back of the chair. He asks me to describe my safe place, I tell him. His voice in response, low. Steady. Soothing. Breathe in, and out. He moves through each limb of my body, asking me to tense and relax each one. Again. And again. Heavy now, full. Let your mind go where it wants, where it needs to.

My safe place dissolves. Other things come into the foreground. Images sharpen. My mind cycles, swims against them, tries to reject them. A room. A bed. Darkness, the outline of trees dancing manic patterns on the ceiling. The feeling of being watched, a dark shadow behind me. Beside me. Breath on my neck. The bed depresses as the shadow lies next to me. Too close. It doesn't speak, it moves all around me. Over me. Bad. Worse. Mike's voice is far away now, I can hardly hear what he's saying. I keep going back to a place I don't want to, the room opposite mine, the sound of children crying. You laughing.

He asks me what else I can see, or hear. A pair of yellow eyes glowing in the dark, I tell him. A black cat, the size of a human, a sentry by my bed, sent to watch, to keep me there. Extending and retracting its claws.

'I don't like it there, I want to leave.'

Mike's voice, clearer now, tells me to go back to my safe place. Walk towards it, he says. So I do. The hollow in the old oak tree, behind our house. I used to climb into it, the heart of the tree, when you worked weekends and didn't always take me with you, watch the way the light changed over the field. Crimson and orange.

Safe.

'When you feel ready, open your eyes, Milly.'

I stay still for a minute or two. A feeling of wet under my chin. I open my eyes, look down at the cushion, tie-dyed with tears, the velvet mottled. I look over at Mike. His eyes are closed, he pinches his fingers above the bridge of his nose, massages a little. Making the switch from psychologist to foster dad. He opens his eyes when I speak.

'I must have been crying.'

'Sometimes remembering does that to us.'

'Isn't there another way?'

Mike shakes his head, sits forward in his seat, says, 'The only way out is through.'

I open Saskia's present when I get back to my room. The first thing I see inside the small square box is: gold. A chain with a name. Milly, my new name, not Annie. I run my fingers over the edges of the letters, the sharp points, wondering how much a name can change a person, if at all.

I finish off an essay for French and am about to do some drawing when I hear Phoebe's door open, close again, footsteps on the stairs as if she's dumped her stuff and gone back down. I follow a few minutes later. I want to see if Saskia is home so I can thank her.

I find her in the snug with Phoebe, a cosy room full of soft sofas, a cinema screen mounted on the wall. The TV's on but Saskia flicks it off when I come in. She cradles a drink against her chest. The clink of ice cubes, a heavy short glass, crystal. A slice of lime. Phoebe's slouched over her phone, doesn't look up.

'Hi, Milly, are you feeling better? Mike said you had a migraine.'

'Much better, thanks, and thank you for my present.'

I hold up the necklace, she smiles, foggy. She likes her drink strong and, when it's mixed with the tablets she takes, lethal. Phoebe looks up, pushes herself off the sofa, walks over to me.

'Let me see,' she says, but doesn't wait for me to show her, grabs the chain from my hand. Saskia untucks her legs, puts the glass down on the low table in front of her, piles and piles of interior design magazines. She's about to stand up, I think, but before she can Phoebe turns towards her and says, 'Unbelievable. Special you said, you had mine made for passing my exams last year. What's she done that's so special?'

'Phoebs, don't. It's a welcome present, it was supposed to make —'

'I know exactly what you meant to do.'

Phoebe turns back to face me, says, 'Don't think you're special, because you're not.' She thrusts the necklace into my chest, shoves past me.

I turn to Saskia and say I'm sorry, but she says it's her fault not mine, then picks up her drink, finishes it, sinks back into the sofa and stares at the blank television screen.

7

The next morning I try to ignore the nerves I feel about
Phoebe, the way she views me as another unwelcome
intruder, the newest on a long list of foster kids. As I go
down the stairs I vow to find a way to make it better, make
it work with her. I pause on the first-floor landing, listen
to the conversation going on between her and Mike.

'Why does she get to miss school again?' she asks. 'Why
don't I?'

It's obvious by the jovial, teasing way Mike responds to
her that Miss Kemp hasn't told him about the poster on my
locker. She must be dealing with it in her own way. Hand-
ling it 'on the quiet'.

I feel through my shirt for the ridges across my ribs. The
familiar pattern of scars hidden high. A language only I
understand. A code, a map. Braille on my skin. Where
I've been, what happened to me there. You hated it when I
cut myself, a filthy disgusting habit you'd say, but try as
I might, I couldn't stop.

Footsteps above me jolt me into the present, I lower my
hand. One floor up, Saskia walks on to the landing, makes
her way down towards me.

'Morning, everything okay?'

A pang in her voice, desperate to be trusted, to do a better job with me than she has with Phoebe. I nod my head.
Withhold. The reality is, most people can't handle the
truth, my truth. A padding sounds across the marble below.

Rosie. She circles a few times, collapses on to the tiles, a shaft of September sun. I watch her breathe. Her scruffy underbelly rises and falls. I think about my dog, Bullet, a Jack Russell we rescued from the pound, another attempt to look normal, and to rid the old house we lived in of rats. They soon moved on, you called him a good boy until he turned his attentions to the cellar. Scratching and sniffing at the door. Instinct told him, he knew what was in there.

He could smell it.

You drowned him in a bucket when I was at school. Left his body rigid, sleek wet fur. I wrapped him in the blanket from his basket, buried him in the garden. I couldn't bring myself to put him in the cellar. Not there.

It took less than a week for the rats to come back.

Saskia smiles, says, I know it's a big day today, let's get a good breakfast into you. I follow her and the scent of her expensive body oil into the kitchen.

The radio is on, the headlines.

You.

The star attraction for all the wrong reasons. It's subtle, but I hear it, the edge in the presenter's voice as she details the charges against you. Saskia and Mike glance at each other. Phoebe doesn't know, but pauses anyway, toast swaying at the entrance to her mouth.

'Psycho bitch, they should hang her,' she says.

A knot in my stomach. I make contact with the nearest thing, swipe it off the counter. A splintering as it hits the slate tiles, a red ooze of jam colours the floor. I kneel down, my hand meets the glass. More red, this time from my finger. There's a scraping of chairs and someone switches off the radio. Sorry, I say. Sorry. Phoebe looks down at me, mouths 'freak' and walks out, I hear Rosie yelp as she passes her.

Mike crouches next to me. We shouldn't have had the news on, we didn't want you to hear that, he says.

Your name. The charges against you, Mummy.

My reality spelled out in public.

I shrug. All I see is red, I'm used to it. The spillages and seepages, how red trickles into the cracks of the floorboards, and no amount of scrubbing erases it. I remember the hours spent in the secure unit, where 'they', the professionals, tried to prepare me for life after you. How to answer questions like where I'm from, what school I used to go to, why I live in a foster family. What they didn't prepare me for, couldn't prepare me for, is how much I look like you. And although you're in the news most days, when the court case is in full swing it'll be worse. So much worse. You will be everywhere.

I will be everywhere.

You're the spit of your mother, they used to say at the women's refuge you worked at. *That's what I'm afraid of*, I replied in my head.

I clear up the mess on the floor. Mike tries to help but I ask him not to, he hands me a plaster for my finger. Have something to eat, Saskia says. Practise what you preach, I want to reply, but instead I say, 'I don't think I can manage breakfast, I'm going to go and brush my teeth.'

Mike says he'll wait for me in the hallway, not to be too long, we need to be at the lawyers' by nine. I hear Phoebe on the phone, laughing, as I pass her room. Relaying the story about me dropping the jam, probably to Izzy or Clondine. And when I'm brushing my teeth I hear your voice: WHO DOES THAT? WHO HANDS IN THEIR MOTHER? I don't answer, I don't know what to say or how I feel about being that person.

When I make my way back downstairs, I pause to tickle Rosie on her tummy, the hair of her coat gingery, bristly. She appreciates the gesture, gentle touch, her tail sweeping the floor.

'She likes you, you know,' Mike says as he approaches.

'I like her.'

'We'll take the Tube I think, it'll be quicker than waiting in traffic.'

We join the throngs of commuters as we reach Notting Hill Gate, head down into the Underground and on to a train. The carriage is busy, full of City workers in suits, jackets off, sleeves rolled up to escape the heat of the Underground, even in September. Life, so different in London, the way people move around together, live so close to each other. No acres of privacy here. Mike and I stand, sandwiched between the crowds, get off at a station called St Paul's, and as soon as we emerge into the open, Mike starts a conversation about the trial, about the options available to me if I have to go to court.

'I've been thinking about it a lot,' he says. 'About the special measures you've been placed under, so you can use a live video link instead of having to go into the courtroom. What do you think about that?'

Futile. That's what I think. I can feel you lining up the guns, loading them. I could say yes to Mike, yes, I'd much rather give evidence from a video link, but he doesn't know the feelings I live with every day. That even though I'm no longer with you, a part of me still wants to please you and indulge my desire to be close to you again, the same room. The last chance I'll get.

I hear Mike say, 'Let's take a left here, avoid the crowds.' We leave the main road and walk down a cobbled alleyway, the change of pace and noise calming. St Paul's Cathedral rises up between the gaps in the buildings. Until today I'd only seen it in pictures. So much more beautiful in real life. I never thought I would like living in a big city, but the density of the buildings, the amount of people, is reassuring. Safe.

'Milly, you didn't answer me. Did you hear what I said?'

'Yeah, I did, sorry, and I get why you think the video link is a good idea, but what if I want to opt out? What if I don't want to use special measures? When June came to see me at the hospital she left me a leaflet. It said I was allowed to do that.'

'You can opt out, but I'm not sure why you'd want to do that?'

I can't tell him, I'm not able to say it. That the person I want to run from is also the person I want to run to. So instead I tell him it's because, for once, I want to choose. I want to be the one making a decision involving me.

'I appreciate where you're coming from but I'm not sure I agree, especially after this morning. You were very upset when the headlines came on.'

'It was more of a shock than anything, the jam slipped through my fingers, an accident.'

'I know, but still, we want to protect you.'

He can't. Nobody can. There's a game being played, a secret head-to-head. No referee. My only chance to break free is if I go to court.

'I'll be sixteen soon, Mike. I'm not a kid any more. I want the chance to do this, to feel brave, to walk away knowing I managed to stand up in court and be questioned, knowing that she was there too.'

'I need to think about it some more, Milly, but what I

45

can say is that you're doing very well, better than anyone could have hoped.'

'So in reality I should be able to manage to go to court.'

We stop at the end of the alleyway, where it rejoins the main road, the noise from the traffic apparent again. He turns to face me. I give him eye contact – I can, when necessary, just not for long.

He nods, cognitive wheels rotating. A spit inside his head.

'We'll talk to the lawyers about it today. I can see your point of view but everybody has to be in agreement on this one and, to be honest, I'm not sure June will be. But if it's any consolation, I'll talk to her, at least help her see it from your point of view as well, and we'll go from there. Okay?'

'Okay. Thank you.'

Got him, just where I want him.

We enter the reception of the lawyers' offices through a large set of revolving doors, an atrium flooded with light from a dome-shaped glass ceiling. June's there already, smiles as she greets us. When I met her at the unit she said, in a thick Northern Irish accent, we want what's best for you. You don't even know me, I wanted to reply.

'Hi, guys, did you dander your way here okay?'

'Yeah, no problem at all,' Mike replies.

'Hi, Milly, nice to see you again, it's been a while. You okay?'

I nod. Look up at the offices surrounding us, floor after floor, a corporate cake, no cherry on the top. People in suits, neutral looks on their faces. Masks. A sense of purpose in the air, movement, shoes tapping across the floor, also marble. A security guard monitors the turnstiles as identification cards on lanyards round necks are removed and swiped. So many decisions made here, so many lives changed. Soon it will be your life. And mine.

'Milly.'

'Milly. June's talking to you.'

'Sorry.'

'I was just explaining to Mike that the courthouse, which is called the Old Bailey, isn't far from here. You're to use the underground car park if you're called to attend the trial at any point.'

'Why?'

'Just a precaution really.'

She looks at Mike. He looks back. The world turns on a million different looks. Glances. I work hard to decipher them, harder than most. My psychologist at the unit enlightened me. You may have a compromised ability to read emotions, he said. He meant: my mind does not function the same way an average person's does. So I read textbooks, watch people on TV and in the street. I practise. Leaps and bounds, improvement can always be made. 'Average' is not a word I like.

'It's nothing to worry about, it's just sometimes there can be a bit of a crowd outside when there's big trials going on. Some real eejits, mostly just looking for trouble.'

'People want to see her, don't they?' I ask.

June places her hand on my forearm, I move it away. Mike nods, he understands.

'Sorry,' she says. 'And yes, people will want to see her but it's also a way of protecting you. Even though the press aren't allowed to mention you by name or use any photographs, you never know.'

'Shall we make a move,' Mike says. 'It's almost nine.'

'We should, you're right, the lawyers are waiting. Must

47

be about time for a cup of tea as well, maybe even a choccy bicky if we're lucky. You fancy that, Milly?'

I nod, fancying the idea of shoving one down her throat more.

We take the lift to level -2, the bowels of the building. Quiet. We won't be disturbed. I'm disturbed enough already, they think. June shows us into a room, two men around a large rectangular table. Long strip lighting, a migraine threatens, will be made worse by the slight flickering from the light furthest away at the back of the room. Coffee- and teacups in the middle of the table, proper cups made out of china, no polystyrene excuses. The detective at the police station where I gave my first statement said it was for safety, you can't smash polystyrene, love.

I remember thinking, no, but you could use the scalding contents.

The men stand up, shake hands with Mike. Crown Prosecutors is their official title. I wonder if they were specially selected, or perhaps they volunteered. Perhaps there was a scrum of volunteers, all keen to be involved in one of the most high-profile cases ever to be tried. Their job is to pursue, and persuade the jury to nail you to the wall. Merely a formality, I've been told. Your ship has sailed. A one-way ticket to jail. Do not pass go, do not collect two hundred. Fucked.

I did that to you.

I don't catch their names, Skinny and Fatty will do, easy to remember.

'Shall we begin?' Skinny says.

June kicks off with an update as to how I'm 'coping' at home, and the adjustment to a new school. Mike chips in, good stuff mainly. Everyone's impressed by how well I'm doing.

'No disturbed sleep?' June asks.

'Not really,' I reply.

Lie.

Mike casts a fleeting look at me, he suspects otherwise, says nothing. Ownership. He'll take the credit for me doing well, *looking* like I'm doing well. I wonder if he'd also take the fall if I turned out just like you.

Fatty moves on to discuss the trial process in detail, says that if need be I'll be brought in the week before to watch my evidence video.

'By then we'll know the angle the defence lawyers plan to come in at – and how to bring them down, of course,' he says.

Leans back in his chair. Pudgy interlocked sausages at the end of his hands, resting on his fat stomach. Smug. Buttons strain in protest. I look away, sickened by his lack of discipline. He continues.

'The jury will be presented with the details of your childhood. They'll be given copies of your medical records, including the extent of your –'

He pauses, the room heavy with words he can't say. I look at him, his turn to struggle with eye contact. He nods slightly, we move on. I don't blame him, a common reaction. I heard the nurses at the hospital discussing my injuries. Out of earshot, they thought. Never seen anything like it, one said, her own mother it was, and she's a nurse would you believe. Yes, another replied, that's why most of the injuries were never reported, dealt with at home, she'll never be able to have kids, you know. You told me I should be thankful, you'd done me a favour. Children were nothing but trouble.

'The final and perhaps most important point to be

discussed is whether or not Milly presents in court,' Skinny says. 'And at some level this may be out of our control due to developments in the last few days.'

'Developments?' June asks.

'There've been noises from the defence camp in regards to certain things they'd like to question Milly on.'

A pounding in my chest. A carrier pigeon, an important message in a small barrel round its neck. Cage door locked, while the others fly free.

'What sort of things?' June asks.

'We're not entirely clear yet, and it's probably not helpful to dwell on it too much until we're sure,' Fatty says.

'Well, it would have been helpful to know about this prior to today,' Mike says, looking first at me then the law-yers. 'It doesn't leave Milly in a very nice position, wondering what it is they want to ask her.'

I have a feeling I know. A bad feeling.

'Agreed,' says June.

'Like I said, it's a new development and at this point they're keeping their cards close to their chest,' Skinny responds.

'Seems like desperate measures to me, given the evidence.'

No, June, not desperate, but the first phase of a plan being exe-cuted by you, Mummy.

'In terms of what it means for Milly,' Skinny responds, 'we should prepare her for the eventuality she'll be cross-examined on her evidence.'

'Mike,' I say.

He looks at me. 'It's okay, it's going to be okay.'

Stomach empty, no breakfast, yet my throat feels full. Swallow. I'm not on trial, you are. That's all I need to remember.

'How likely is it looking?' June asks.

'We're pretty sure the defence will want to go down that route. It'll be the judge, taking into account our recommendations, who makes the final decision, but it's not all doom and gloom,' Skinny replies. 'Milly has the choice of doing it through a video link or – if we think she can handle it – she can go on the stand. There'll be a screen set up so Milly won't be able to see her mother. In my opinion, putting her on the stand can only evoke a favourable response from the jury. Nothing like a kid in court to pull in the sympathy.'

'I don't like the idea of Milly being used as bait,' Mike responds.

'I second that,' June says.

'Like it or loathe it, it's the nature of the court system,' Skinny says. 'And at the end of the day, we all want the same thing.'

Everybody at the table nods but me, I focus on breathing. Calm. On not letting them know I can hear you laughing in my head.

'What about you, Milly? What do you think?' June asks.

Protégée. You loved saying that word. Brave enough. Am I? The lessons you gave me, good enough. Were they? You want them to blame me. YOU WERE THERE TOO, ANNIE. I try to block out your voice, answer June's question.

'Me and Mike have been talking a bit about it and we think by the time the trial starts I'll be strong enough, and that it might actually help if I go into the courtroom.'

'Very sensible attitude,' Skinny says, picking a small scab to the right of his mouth. The sight makes me feel uncomfortable so I look away, turn towards the flickering light, but it makes me feel dizzy and my heart beats faster.

'It all sounds rather gung-ho if you ask me.'

Well we didn't, June, did we?

'We all know what the defence lawyers can be like when they get going,' she continues.

A blockage in my throat, I'd scream if I could. Pins and needles in my feet from pushing them hard into the ground. If only I could tell them why it's so important I go to court. Why I have to play the game with you. I look at Mike, give him eyes enough, ask him to step in. He does.

'Milly and I will work on strategies over the following weeks but in my opinion she does seem to have her head in a reasonable place about this. It might also be useful to view this as an opportunity for closure. A cathartic experience if handled correctly.'

'And if it's not? I'm sorry to play devil's advocate here, but what if it's too difficult for her in the actual moment? What if the defence go hard, try and confuse her, manipulate her into agreeing with their version of events? She feels guilty enough as it is.'

'Hang on, June, I'm not sure it's helpful to talk about Milly's feelings in front of everybody.'

'Sorry, you're right. But we do need to make a decision about this and I think it might be beneficial if we stepped outside to do that. Shall we?'

She gestures to Mike and the lawyers and they leave the room, saying they won't be long. I trace the ripples of scars through my shirt. Count them. Twenty times, or more.

I ask you what happens if I don't want to play, if I say no. Your reply, a scornful voice. YOU'LL ALWAYS WANT TO PLAY, MY LITTLE ANNIE, I MADE YOU THAT WAY.

Finally, they return. Skinny first, then June, followed by Mike. Fatty, gone. An early lunch. And this little piggy always had some.

I hear nothing else apart from Skinny's words.

'We've agreed that if you're called, you'll take the stand.'

But instead of satisfaction, it's a gap I feel, opening up inside me. An empty, lonely place. Nobody can help me now.

A discussion kicks off around how to manage my exposure to press coverage in the run-up to the trial, limit the time I watch the news and listen to the radio. Mike, my monitor. They advise me to keep busy. Some of it I hear, most of it, I don't.

I'm listening to another voice, one that says:

GAME ON, ANNIE.

8

Mike drops me at Wetherbridge just before morning break. He tells me he's proud of me, I thank him, wish I could feel the same. As I sign in at the office I realize I forgot to remind him I'm meeting Miss Kemp after school, so I send him a text while I enjoy the last few minutes of quiet in the locker room. No poster greets me today but when I log on to the school email from my laptop – another present from Mike and Saskia – there's a message from Miss Kemp:

Hi, Milly, really looking forward to our meeting today. Thought we could do some sketching? See you in the art room later.

MK.

MK. I've never known a teacher to sign off with initials before.

The rest of the day is uneventful. Maths, double science and religious studies to end on. When the bell goes, I head up to the art room. I hear their voices before I see them. Nasal and shrill. Mean. Girls. They come down the stairs towards me and I wonder what sort of punishment, if any, MK gave them for the poster. I pause to let them pass, the staircase not wide enough. Phoebe pushes me against the banister.

'Hello, dog-face.'

Dog-face? We were supposed to become sisters. Little women.

'She's waiting for you. So sweet that you got your itty-bitty Miss Kemp to fight your battles.'

'About the necklace, Phoebe, I won't wear it, I feel bad.'

'What's this about a necklace?' Izzy asks.

'Nothing,' Phoebe responds.

'Oh, come on, share,' Izzy says, jabbing her in the stomach.

Depleted. Less hostile, less brave. Embarrassed in front of her friend. I should feel bad for mentioning it now, in front of someone else. I should.

'My stupid fuck-face of a mother bought her one of those gold name necklaces too.'

'The one she had made for you? Did she not have one made for herself as well, so you guys could be matching?'

Phoebe nods. I try to say sorry, but she tells me to shut up.

'Uh-oh, dearest Mummy let you down again, has she?'

'Fuck off, Iz.'

'Chill out, who needs mothers anyway when we have each other?'

They laugh and continue down the stairs to the next landing. I say nothing, but I want to say, I do.

I need a mother.

Izzy stops, looks up at me, asks, 'Had any strange phone calls recently?'

My hand moves towards my phone in my blazer pocket.

'I take it by the silence that's a no then. Well, strap in, I'm sure it won't be long.'

More sniggers and laughter.

Salt in the wound. Stings. As I look down at their beautiful faces I remember a story I read. A Native American tale where the Cherokee tells his grandson there's a battle between two wolves in all of us. One is evil, the other

56

good. The boy asks him, which wolf wins? The Cherokee tells him, the one you feed. Their faces become targets as I look at them. I'm tempted to open my mouth, saliva and spit across the make-up on their faces. Dolls. A biscuity smell of fake tan hangs in the air. Izzy makes a V with her fingers, shoves her tongue through them. Phoebe does the same. Bad thoughts in my head. A door opens in the corridor below, prompts them to move. I check my phone as I head up the remaining stairs to MK's room, no calls.

When I arrive there are two easels set up opposite each other. Two stools, two boxes of charcoal. Two of everything.

'Hey,' she says. 'Welcome! Ready to do some sketching?'

I nod, place my bag and blazer down. She asks me if I'd like a glass of water.

'No thank you.'

'Have you worked with charcoal before?'

'A little bit.'

'Good, grab a seat at one of the easels.'

Her hands are flighty, move quickly, as if the weight of the rings would be too heavy if they remained stationary for more than a split second. She sits down opposite me.

'Any idea what you'd like to draw?'

Yes. But I don't think people would approve.

'Not really, I don't mind.'

'How about we sketch the figure over there on the table, it's by a sculptor called Giacometti, or I've got some perfume in my bag, the bottle's an interesting shape.'

Her perfume. That's what it is. Familiar. Fresh sprigs of lavender cut from our garden, by you.

'The figure is fine,' I reply.

'Good choice, I'll grab it.'

She moves with fluidity, the tribal beads she wears

leaving a wake of noise with each step. Her hair piled up in a messy bump, secured by a clip with some kind of Asian pattern on it. She reminds me of something from a *National Geographic* magazine – a cross between a messy geisha and a tribal high priestess. We begin sketching at the same time, in tune somehow, our hands synchronized, reach for the charcoal. She asks me how things have been so far, I tell her fine.

'Fine as in really fine, or as in could be better but you don't want to say?'

'A bit of both maybe.'

Sweep. Dust. A head on the page, I wonder if she started at the top too.

'Art's an excellent therapy, you know.'

I feel the prickles advance. Half-built walls live inside me, erected fully in minutes if I feel a threat of exposure. 'Therapy'. Why would she say that? A need-to-know basis, Mike said. Ms James, the headmistress at school, and Sas and I, that's it. Nobody else knows about your mother. I look over my easel at her. No make-up, a natural blush. Peaches and cream. She looks up, smiles, gentle crinkles and creases forming round her eyes. I bet she smiles, laughs, a lot.

'How's it going over there?'

'Good, thanks.'

The head has a body now, thin as a whip like the one you used, even though I said no.

'How have things been with the girls?'

Worse than ever.

'Not too bad, I suppose.'

'You suppose?'

'I have a feeling I won't fit in very well here.'

'It can be tough, that's for sure. The girls here are smart and streetwise, most of them have grown up in London their whole lives. I've seen it before, everybody new gets a bit of a rough ride which is what guidance teachers are for, and lucky for me, I got you! Now, are you ready to show me your drawing?'

'I think so, yes.'

She wipes her hands on the damp cloth by her side, stands up and walks over to my easel, makes an appreciative whistling noise, says, boy oh boy, your old headmistress was right.

'Such incredible use of shading, the statue looks like it's moving, walking off the page. Would you mind very much if I kept it? I'd like to show the Year Eights, they're working on figure sketches at the moment.'

'Sure, of course, if you think it's good enough.'

I'm about to unclip the paper but she tells me to stop, that I've forgotten something.

'Oh, sorry.'

'An artist must always sign their work.'

I look up at her, she winks, nudges my shoulder, and I don't feel weird or uncomfortable in the same way I did when June touched me. I sign it, but need to be more careful in future – I almost signed it Annie.

I'm about to leave when she says, 'Don't worry about the girls, I'm keeping a close eye on them. I've had them in here tidying up and scrubbing palette pots. They seem to feel sorry for what they did so I'm sure it's the last we'll hear of it. Why don't you grab a roll of paper on the way out and a box of charcoal, keep up the sketching at home?'

A warm feeling as I leave, the good wolf. Feasted.

A stillness fills the corridors, I don't have to rush or

worry about avoiding the rest of the girls. I head to my locker to pick up a folder I forgot and get halfway across the school courtyard when my phone rings. A number I don't recognize.

A flash of Izzy's face sneering at me when she said, 'Had any strange phone calls yet?'

I shouldn't answer, but curiosity gets the better of me. Curiosity killed the.

'Hello.'

'Is that Milly?'

A deep voice. Muffled.

'Who is this?' I reply.

'I'm ringing about the advert.'

'What advert?'

'The postcard.'

'What postcard?'

'Oh, come on, love, no need to be shy.'

'How did you get this number?'

'From the advert, I told you. Look, I'm not being funny but are you for real or not?'

'I might be.'

'You like playing games, do you?' he asks.

His voice. Different, more urgent. I recognize what it means.

'Depends,' I reply.

'On what?'

'If I get to win or not.'

I hang up, stare at the phone for a few seconds, leave the courtyard. Although it was warm on the Tube this morning, the evening wind has changed in the past couple of weeks, brushes over my hands with a cool edge. I put my phone in my blazer pocket, too much to hold with the folder and the roll of paper MK gave me. I feel a vibration against my thigh, a message. I don't stop to read it, in a few minutes I'll be home. When I reach the turning into my road, I pull my phone out from my pocket, an unknown number again.

My cocks hard and ready arrange to meet

I read it again, unsure if the content or the fact it's written without punctuation offends me more. Uncouth. The message disappears off the screen as a call comes in. I recognize the number this time, the same one as before. I can't help but answer. Fun, almost.

'Yes?'

'Did you hang up on me?'

I pause at the corner, lean into the wall, rest my heavy school rucksack up and off my shoulders.

'Maybe.'

'Are you in your school uniform now?'

'How do you know I go to school?'

'I could tell from the picture – do you wear a skirt or one of those little dresses?'

I can hear the arousal in his voice, obvious to me. I've always wondered if it sounds different in a man than a woman. It doesn't.

'When can we meet? I pay well.'

I hang up. Two nil, loser. I enjoy the power, being desired. I turn into my road, hear someone whistle. Morgan. She uses her fingers like a builder might, or a dog-walker calling her dog. I smile and she nods at me, calls me over then buries her mouth into the zip of her tracksuit so only the top part of her face is visible. She holds something in one of her hands. I walk over. Her eye is less bruised than before but I notice as she brings her mouth out of her top that her lips are chapped and bloody. She chews on them as if they are food. An appetizer.

'Hi.'

She doesn't reply, turns her head to the side, picks at her lips, peels a bit of skin off them. Fresh blood when she turns back as if she's eaten a berry, a more appetizing appetizer. She licks the blood away, wipes the back of her sleeve across her mouth. I can see the thing in her hand is a postcard, but I can't see what of.

'I'm just back from school.'

She shrugs.

'Your eye looks better.'

'Till the next time, yeah.'

'What happened?'

'Walked into a door, that's what my mum always says anyway.' A smirk on her face.

And what Mummy says goes, right?

'You said your name was Milly, yeah?'

'Yes.'

'I found something I think belongs to you, it's got your name and your photo on it. M-I-L-L-Y.'

She sounds out the letters, releases them slowly from her sore lips with concentration.

'Why are you sounding it out like that?'

'Fuck off all right, I'm dyslexic.'

A hurt look passes over her face. I look away, ashamed I caused it.

'Anyway, you don't need to know how to read properly to work this out.'

She hands me the card. A professional job, laminated, quality colour. I think about how it was made, handed around a printing shop perhaps, overweight guys spluttering into mugs of tea as I'm passed back and forth.

'Where did you get it from?'

'Found it last night in the phone box, down on the right by the arches near Ladbroke Grove. My phone's broken and my mum hasn't got any credit on hers.'

I know where she means. Amongst the dirt and grime, piss and chewing gum, a collection of adverts live. Me. A new face, added to the bill. Roll up roll up, a tasty newcomer. A gallery of boobs, open mouths, weird grotesque looks on the women's faces. And now, a schoolgirl. The image, the same one used on the poster left on my locker. New words.

SCHOOLGIRL MILLY 'DTF' READY TO SUCK COCK, CALL NUMBER BELOW

The science-block toilets. Izzy. 'I won't ask again.' My phone vibrates, a buzzing from inside my left pocket, I enjoy a brief moment of how popular feels. Hungry lambs at a teat, enough is never enough.

'No offence, but you don't look the type.'

'I'm not.'

'What's it all about then?'

'Someone's idea of a joke.'

'You must have pissed them right off, it's a pretty sick joke.'

'It's a couple of the girls from school, and the girl I live with.'

'What, that snotty blonde bitch?'

She points towards our house, I look over my shoulder.

'Yeah, her.'

The driveway obscures most of the windows but two or three look out on to the street. I'm hit by an urgency to keep Morgan a secret.

'Has anyone called you?' she asks.

'Somebody just did.'

'Fuck. What are you going to do to get her back?'

I'll think of something.

'Not sure, probably just let it go. How long do you reckon the postcard was up for?'

'Maybe a day or something, I don't know. You just moved here, didn't you?'

I nod, reply, 'They're my foster family.'

'We were almost in care for a bit when my mum was sent down but our nana came and looked after us.'

'So your mum's out now?'

'Yeah, she was only in for a few weeks. Something stupid she helped my uncle with.'

She picks at her lips again. I resist the urge to slap her hand away, tell her to stop. She pushes her body off the wall, stands up. I ask her if she wants to hang out some time. Maybe, she replies. Suspicious. That's good, I want to tell her. Safer that way.

'We could meet at the bottom of my garden. The blue door in the close takes you into it, it's usually locked but I could open it. My room's the one with the balcony.'

'Why are you so keen to hang out?'

'Dunno. It's not easy being the new girl, especially with a foster sister like mine.'

She nods. I get the impression she's lonely too.

'What do you reckon? Do you fancy it?' I ask her again.

'Like I said, maybe. You want us to meet in your garden so no one knows we're friends, isn't it?'

'It's not that, it's to do with the blonde bitch I live with. Your words not mine.'

We both smile when I say it.

'She'd find a way to ruin it, tell her dad or something,' I explain.

'Bet she would, silly cow.'

I need something to close the deal. Gifts open doors, trust comes easier afterwards, I watched you do it a hundred times with the kids at the refuge. THINK, ANNIE, THINK. Your voice in my head. The phone thinks for me, vibrates again in my pocket. I ask Morgan if she's any good with them, take it out, show her.

'I'm all right.'

'What am I supposed to do now that I'm getting calls from the advert?'

'Don't know, change the number?'

'I can't, I'd have to ask my foster dad, he'd figure something was up.'

'Chuck it?'

'It's brand new, it'd be crazy to throw it away. I could tell him I lost it but he'd be pretty angry I think.'

'Who cares, they must have a shitload of money, what's a stupid phone to them.'

'True, but I still feel bad about binning it. You said your phone was broken, maybe you could borrow mine for a bit, get the number changed or something.'

'Nah, it doesn't feel right, I don't even know you.'

'It means we'd be able to stay in touch though, if we did want to hang out.'

'And I wouldn't have to do anything for it?'

'No, nothing. Like I said, you'd be helping me out.'

She chews on her lip some more, stares down at her feet, then looks up and says, okay, deal. She takes it, says she'll find a way to let me know when she's sorted a new number, then asks me what to do with the postcard.

'Was it the only one?'

'Only one that I saw.'

'Do what you like with it, burn it for all I care.'

She nods, and walks away. I watch her go, pleased with myself. Your lessons, your voice, helpful to me. Sometimes.

The house is quiet when I open the door, unlocked, so somebody must be home, likely Saskia, she always forgets to lock the door behind her. The radiator next to the shoe cubby releases a whispering sound, the effort required to keep the entrance porch warm exhausting for its ancient pipes. I notice a pair of trainers on the floor I don't recognize, too large for a woman.

I take off my shoes and dump my stuff at the bottom of the stairs. Rosie looks up at me with half-closed eyes, too comfy to rise out of her basket to greet me, a vague thump of the tail. Dinner is plated, left out on the kitchen counter. Three in a line. Sevita knows better than to leave anything for 'Miss Saskia', which means both Mike and Phoebe are still out. I take the chance to switch on the radio while the stew is heating up in the microwave, see if I can hear anything, but the headlines are over. I eat fast, hoping to avoid Phoebe, and after I put my plate in the dishwasher I head to Mike's study, knock on the door, make sure he's not home. No answer. I use a Post-it note from the block on the table next to the alcove, write 'Dear Mike, I'm so sorry but I've lost my phone, I can't find it anywhere. What should I do?'

I stick it on the middle of his study door, at eye level, so he can't miss it. A neon-pink apology, and a secret fuck you to Phoebe. I want to get a new phone as soon as possible so Morgan and I can stay in touch. I notice the door to the basement is open as I pass it, it leads to the laundry and the gym. I have a quick look to make sure Sevita isn't down there, then close it, wishing there was a lock.

I check from my balcony if I'm right about the gate leading into the garden being hidden from the house. I am. I'm about to come inside when I hear the whistle, a small figure in the close, waving at me. She does something after that with her hands. A spark, another, a lighter being lit, followed by a lick of flame. Impossible to see from this distance, but I know it's the postcard she's burning. When it becomes too hot to hold she drops it on to the ground, makes a swiping motion with her hands, job done, and jogs back up the close towards the street.

I let down my guard, fall asleep too fast. You come to congratulate me. Remind me if it hadn't been for your lessons, I'd never have got Morgan to trust me. I wake up crying.

Up eight. Up another four.
The door on the right.

Put the trousers on.

Put the shirt on.

Do as you're told.

Dress up. Your favourite game.

The boys dressed as boys, the girls did too.

Life-size, walking, talking dolls to play with. Discard when bored.

How special you look as a boy, Annie.

Come closer, let Mummy see.

9

Saskia offers to drive me and Phoebe to school this morning, noticing that as well as my usual load, I have to carry
a large portfolio case for art in which I'll store my work for
this term. Phoebe, dressed in sports gear, says no, plans to
go for a jog before school with two of the other girls who
live close by, reminds them she's staying at Izzy's overnight. Mike shouts to her when she's putting her shoes on
in the porch, make sure you eat something for breakfast. The front door opens, and slams. He tuts, smiling
shortly afterwards.

'I saw the note about losing your phone. Usually I'd say
wait a few days to see if it turns up but I feel better knowing I can get hold of you if needs be. I'll replace it this time,
but please be more careful.'

I ask him to change the number, helps me feel secure. He
says he understands, he'll have it sorted by tonight. I eat a
bowl of cereal while I wait for Saskia to get dressed and,
when she's ready, we head out to her car, a soft-top Mini. I
load the portfolio case into the boot, just about fits. An area
of London where style trumps practicality. Appearance
matters. Air kisses, as knives are simultaneously slid into
backs. Twisted.

'Ready?' she asks, climbing into the driving seat.

I nod, annoyed by the way she said 'ready' in an overly
chirpy manner. Scratch the perfectly applied foundation
on her skin, weakness lurks. A cardboard cut-out of a

mother. She hits the accelerator too hard, the car jerks across the gravel with protest. I want to say, relax, I don't bite. Well I do, but I won't. She's wary of me. Female intuition maybe. She can't forget who I am, who I've come from. Belong to. When she thinks I'm distracted, and I won't notice, I see her looking.

I notice.

'This is nice,' she says as we turn out of the drive.

'Yes,' I reply, looking for Morgan.

'How's school going?'

'Busy, a lot to take in.'

'Mike tells me you're interested in art.'

'I like drawing.'

'I was always terrible at art, terrible at most things to be honest. Not like you, very smart I hear.'

'I'm not really sure about the smart bit, but thanks. Can I ask you something?'

'Sure, fire away.'

'What do you do during the day when Mike's at work and we're at school?'

'Lots of different things, I suppose.'

'Like what, if you don't mind me asking?'

I turn to face her, she clears her throat, looks away. An involuntary response to being in the hot seat, with something to hide, secretly she's glad the school run's only a couple of minutes.

'Bits and bobs really. Online shopping for the house.'

Yes, which the housekeeper puts away.

'Sometimes I get together with the other mums to discuss school stuff and before you know it the day's gone and the house is full of you guys again.'

'You forgot yoga. You love it, don't you?'

72

'Yes, that's right, silly of me to forget. I like it very much, do it most days.'

I wait a few seconds, then say, 'And your teacher, you really like him.'

The creamy complexion of her face changes colour. Reddens. A tightening round her lips. She removes her left hand from the gear stick, flicks her nose a few times. Deceit. I'm not the only one withholding.

'Yes, he's excellent,' she replies.

'Was he over last night by any chance?'

She looks at me. I read her thought process easily. Surely not, she's wondering. The house was empty, wasn't it? She turns away before answering.

'As a matter of fact, he was. I ordered a new mat and he decided to drop it in. He was passing by, I think.'

The pitch of her voice. Up a fraction. The car comes to a halt, traffic lights add pain. Hers. Pleasure, mine. Then guilt. I don't know why I'm taunting her, why I'm enjoying it.

I tell Saskia that was nice of him, to deliver the mat. She nods, wary of what else is to come, but I stop there. I don't tell her that before I closed the door to the basement last night, I heard noises. I don't tell her I went down the steps to the gym and saw her being fucked on the floor by a man half her age. Slut. I don't tell her because secrets, when handled carefully, can be useful.

'This is about as close as I can get,' she says and pulls the car into the kerb outside the newsagent across the road from school.

'It's fine, I'll just grab my stuff from the boot.'

As I turn to open the car door, I see you on the front cover of a newspaper outside the shop. Saskia hurries me, says she's holding up traffic. I climb out, shut the door, collect my portfolio case from the boot and, once I close it, Saskia toots her horn and drives off. I take as long as possible to load my things from the pavement into my arms, my eyes on you. Somebody behind me says, could you be any more in the way? I gather everything up and head for the zebra crossing. Tall orange lollipops, a stream of pupils in uniform.

I make my way to the common room, usually a place much like the 'middle corridor' I avoid, but a compulsory meeting for our year group's school play, *Lord of the Flies*, is scheduled there first thing this morning. I open the door. Phoebe is the first person I see, already changed from her running gear into uniform. A handful of other girls lounge on the beanbags and sofas. Most of them don't look up as I come in, heads bent over phones. Fingers tap. Scroll. Up. Down. The kidnapping of women and children in Nigeria is not what they read about. They obsess over the small things, the insignificant things. The celebrity break-ups. Make-ups. The babies. Divorce. Who cheated on who. She deserved it anyway, stupid cow. Comments thrown back and forth. Fingers pick up speed. Tap. Double tap. Tap again. Un-tap, because they change their minds. Fickle like that.

I leave my art case by the door and without thinking pick up a newspaper from the table closest to me and take a seat. My heart rate increases when I realize you're on the front cover of this one too. Now is not the time to enjoy you, enjoy looking at you. I open the paper, doesn't matter which page, can't concentrate on the words anyway. A minute or so later Phoebe moves from her position on the window seat, walks towards me, grabs it from my hands. Shield. Armour. Gone. She has you, your face, in her right hand.

'Thanks, dog-face, you know how much I love to keep up with the news.'

She flops into the chair opposite me. Her school skirt, rolled over at the waist, sits shorter than it should, reveals the remnants of a summer tan on her toned legs. Ankle-length socks, we'll be switching to tights next week, I bet she'll find a way to make them alluring. She draws up her legs, rests her feet on the table between us, knickers visible, newspaper on her thighs. Ink scribbled below her knee, a doodle of a love heart next to an old scar. Oval in shape. Looking at it reminds me of you, you loved to leave your mark on me. Conquered and claimed. I stare when I think about you, it's a problem I have. Layers of thoughts, pinball speed in my head.

Don't realize I'm doing it.

'Like staring at girls' knickers, do you?'

I look away, some of the girls laugh, others busy, engaged in their shallow cyber graves. Phoebe goes back to reading and out of the corner of my eye I see her shaking her head and when she says, fuck, I know she's talking about you.

'Clonny.'

'Yeah?'

'There's some more stuff about that psycho bitch that killed those kids.'

'Fuck, really? What does it say?'

'Something about a playground. Come here, I'll show you.'

Clondine heaves herself off a beanbag, crawls towards her. My body reacts. Panic. Cold sweat. The back of my neck.

'Shall I read it out loud?' Phoebe asks.

'Yeah, go on,' Clondine replies.

I swallow, try to. Gremlin fingers block my throat. A nasty taste. Don't be sick, can't be. Not here.

Interest is piqued. Girl by girl, bees to honey. They slide into the chairs next to Phoebe, peer over shoulders, she knows how to work a crowd.

'Forty-eight-year-old Ruth Thompson was a popular member of staff at the women's refuge where she worked. Employed as a Nurse Counsellor, she was the main point of contact for the scores of frightened women and their children who were in hiding, often fleeing dangerous and violent partners. Little did they know they had met a person equally, if not more evil in her. Thompson was arrested in July this year and charged with nine counts of child murder, said to have been committed over a period of ten years, from 2006 to 2016. New details emerging claim these murders were carried out in a bedroom she called the playground at her home in Devon. Following her arrest, the bodies of eight children were discovered in the cellar of the house and a ninth found in the so-called playground. The victims are thought to be between the ages of three and six years old. Thompson lived in this property with a teenage child of her own who is said to have provided crucial evidence in the case against her.'

'What the fuck? She was a mum? Oh my god, imagine living with her.'

'Yeah, you'd be thinking you'd be next the whole time.'

'The playground? What a sick fucker. I wonder what else is still to come out.'

The rest of the words Phoebe reads – Abuse – Peephole – Secrets – merge into one as I think about what Aimee said – 'you'd be thinking you'd be next the whole time'.

I used to think that too, about being next. But you couldn't, could you? Not because you love me, not because you would have been devastated, bereft without me. You

76

kept me alive because you needed me. I was part of your disguise.

When Phoebe's finished reading, silence. Breath held, exhaled. F-bombs drop. French Marie cuts the atmosphere, says, maybe our mothers are not so bad after all, hey? Heads nod. Bit by bit the pack splits, back to their original seats. Heads down, fingers tap. Quick, five minutes, gone. Catch up. The world can change in the blink of a social media eye. Not Phoebe, her head isn't down, she's looking at me. All I can think is, I'm the spit of you, and somehow she's worked it out.

'What are your thoughts, dog-face? Reckon she's guilty?'

I know she is.

'It's up to the court to decide.'

'You don't sound very bothered, or perhaps you're into fucked-up stuff as well, we all know foster kids aren't right in the head.'

I turn my face to the side, ashamed by an urge to cry, but this provokes her further. She hates being ignored.

'Such a smart-arse, aren't you, told Dad you lost your phone, did you? How about I tell him exactly what kind of extra-curricular activities you're into? Schoolgirl down to fuck, isn't that what the advert said?'

The way she says it. Drips off her tongue, from those lips. Glistening. Divine. I turn back to face her as do most of the heads in the room. Clondine sniggers as she films, her phone held in the air. Standard. It'll be played, replayed, edited. Music added. Anything to make it worthy of views on Facebook or Instagram. The bell sounds, first period. Somebody asks where the fuck Miss Mehmet is. A sharp throbbing sensation, my hand in my blazer pocket, I don't need to look to know I've peeled away the skin on my thumb, enough to make it bleed. I know what time it is from the bell but I look at the clock anyway, away from Phoebe's eagle eyes. The cushion she throws pounds me on the side of my face. I jump, nerves on edge after hearing her read about you, and the fact you had a child too.

Me.

We're about to clear out when Miss Mehmet arrives, flounces in, announces who's playing which part in the play and asks for volunteers for backstage and scenery painting. The auditions were held on Tuesday when I was off with the migraine but she asks me to take the job of prompt, goes on to remind us to use the Year Eleven forum as an arena for brainstorming ideas.

'Get together to practise your lines, girls, immerse yourself in your characters. Eat, sleep and drink this play, I expect nothing but the best from all of you.'

The common room empties. I stay behind, smooth out the wrinkles Phoebe left after reading you out loud. I place you on top of the bookshelf, the idea of your face being scribbled on or used as a coaster. Too much. A minute after I leave I return, rip out the page with your picture on and place it in the front pocket of my school bag.

Third period, I log on to the forum. A private place, a private space, a show of trust from the headmistress for the Year Elevens. Password protected by a nominated individual, none other than queen bee, Phoebe Newmont. Quotes and poems. Homework. And videos, now. The most recent one uploaded, 'Dog-face gets cushioned.' The responses are mainly 'crying with laughter' emojis. Izzy commented, 'More please!!'

I tried so hard not to believe the things you used to say – it's just me and you, Annie, nobody else will want you. I'd agree, say, yes, you're right, of course. Programmed to obey. But late in the night when the threat of your visiting shadow kept me awake, I'd reject your words in my head. Clinging on to the thought that, one day, I could be liked and accepted for being me. Whoever. Whatever that might be. But currently I don't stand a chance, Phoebe's seen to that. Quickly decided not only was I someone she didn't like, but someone that nobody else should either. Powerful, like you.

Hurt. It does, to be Phoebe's target, but it is at some level inclusion. A learning opportunity, one I am hungry for. I'm my own teacher now though your lessons still ring loud in my head. I remember one weekend, helping at your work. I played with the children while you tended to their mothers. One of the women commented on me, called me beautiful. Striking. In the car on the way home you told me, beauty gives a person power.

And camouflage.

It has for me, you said, and it will for you.

I asked you what you meant. It's nature, you replied. Beauty blinds, draws people in. A brightly coloured tree frog, a spider that smiles. The beautiful shade of blue on its head distracts its prey. The web, sticky. Thick. The prey realizes too late. Realizes what, Mummy? You smiled, pinched my thigh, hard, and said – there's no escape.

Your voice, the way you told stories. Captivating, yet terrifying. I remember thinking I didn't want to blind people or draw them in so they couldn't escape.

I didn't want to be like you.

When I check my computer this morning the news is full to the brim of you. Snippets of information leaked and gobbled up by journalists.

One of the articles reads:

The jury are expected to hear evidence not only from the mother of Daniel Carrington, the last child found dead at Thompson's home, but also from a forensic expert who will answer questions both on his death and the crime scene, the room in Thompson's house of horrors that she called the playground. It's unclear at present if this is a normal part of the proceedings or if the forensic expert has been called upon at the request of the defence. Thompson is currently being held in Low Newton Prison and the trial date is yet to be released.

I wish I could rationalize it in my mind. That the reason the defence want to focus on Daniel's death is because it's the most recent and the evidence is fresh. But I know you better than that. It's you. You've told them to focus their efforts there because you know it'll hurt me the most. I knew Daniel from the refuge. Him and his mum. I think about her all the time, and the other mums. How they must have felt when they realized what you'd done. Who they'd given their children to. Monsters for husbands, but in you, something worse. You'll be thinking about it too, remembering it in a different way though. A way that feeds your penchant for the macabre, enjoying all the buzz surrounding you, seeing how far your lies can reach. I think about the jury too, who they'll be, what kind of people they'll be. And how sorry I feel for them. The things they'll hear, the images they'll be shown. Months it'll take, maybe longer, for them to stop seeing. Imagining. If ever.

The picture the press use, I don't know where they got it from, I've never seen it before. The public will look at your face, into your eyes, and say, look at her, you can tell she's evil, gives me the creeps she does. You won't care, you believe in your beauty, your likeability, even still. The men and women in uniform who guard you, some of them will forget, discuss the weather with you. Maybe even share a joke. You, charming.

The interest from professionals, the many who'll want to interview you, scan images of your brain in an attempt to decode you, will only grow as more details emerge. Female killers who operate alone (yes I was there, but still), are rare. Then there's the others, like the ones you invited for my birthday, lurking, creeping in the shadows. Admiration for you. Pen pals, perhaps even a future marriage proposal, or two. The queen of an underworld nobody wants to acknowledge exists. Ordinary people. Extraordinary evil inside. The brain of a psychopath is different from most, I've weighed up my chances. Eighty per cent genetics, twenty per cent environment.

Me.
One hundred per cent fucked.

I'm glad it's the weekend, no school to worry about. My first whole week over. Survived. Mike left a new phone outside my door on Thursday night. I reach down, unplug it from charging. When I get up and part the curtains to the balcony door, the sky is clear and blue. In the next few weeks when October arrives the sun will sit lower in the sky. When I was very little, three maybe four, I used to like the darkness of winter. We'd light the fire in the living room and sometimes toast marshmallows. It wasn't just us at home then, Dad and Luke were there too. I don't like to think about my brother, how he found a way out, left me behind. The feelings, buried deep. It's something you should think about addressing in time, the psychologist at the unit said, but as part of a longer-term therapy plan, and after the trial. I remember watching the way you were with Luke and wishing it was me, a wish I came to regret.

A scrap of paper tucked behind one of the plant pots on the balcony catches my eye. I unlock the door, go out, pick it up. A phone number, the letter M underneath. Clever girl. Risky though, coming so close to the house. I send a text to the number letting her know it's me. She replies instantly, asks if I want to meet up later. Yes, I answer. She tells me to meet her at three at the bottom of the garden, make sure I wear a hoodie. I get back into bed, cocoon myself in the duvet, enjoy the way Morgan's message makes me feel. I didn't have many friends at my old school, the invites to stay over petered out when they weren't reciprocated. Couldn't be.

I sleep peacefully, feel rested for once, and hungry. I look for Rosie but her basket by the radiator in the entrance hallway is empty and I remember Mike said he sometimes takes her to work with him. More attention than at home.

There's a note on the kitchen table. 'Checked in on

you – FAST ASLEEP!! Text me and Sas your new number please. I'll be at work all day but Sas is around.'

I grab a bowl of cereal, eat it standing up against the warmth of the Aga. I hear the front door open, the antique bell above it sounds and whoever it is goes straight up the stairs.

'Hello?'

But they don't answer, so I go into the hallway. A handbag dumped on the floor, contents spilling out. Saskia. I walk over to it, her purse visible on the top, forced open by the receipts in it. She's a buyer, makes her feel better, for a bit. I'm about to walk away when I see something poking out from the card section in the purse. I take a closer look then go back into the kitchen to tidy away my breakfast things. When I hear footsteps on the landing above I move into the hallway again, make sure we arrive at the same time.

'Hi, I didn't realize you were down here. Did you enjoy your lie-in?' she asks.

A yoga mat slung over her shoulder, kept snug in a handmade silk bag, a present from Mike no doubt, or Benji perhaps, her teacher.

'Yes thank you.'

'What are you up to? If you're interested, you could come to yoga with me?'

Legs, thin like a locust's, shiny in Lycra pulled tight up her crotch. Vagina lips. Outlined. Shaved, probably. She's not shy.

'No thanks, I've got loads of schoolwork to do – everybody seems so ahead at Wetherbridge.'

'I wouldn't worry, you'll soon catch up. Will you be all right on your own? I can stay if you like?'

'No, it's fine.'

'I'll be back in about an hour and a half if you fancy doing something then?'

'I think I'm meeting a friend.'

'Somebody from school?'

'Yes.'

She looks at a watch on her wrist that doesn't exist. Keen to leave.

'I should go,' she says.

Halfway out the door she is, when I call to her.

'Saskia.'

'Yes?'

'I don't like to ask, I know you and Mike have already been so kind, but would I be able to have some money, in case I want to buy a hot chocolate or something?'

'Sure, of course, let me grab my purse. We should sort out an allowance for you, Phoebe has one. I'll speak to Mike tonight.'

I walk towards her in the porch.

'Will twenty do?'

I nod.

'Here you go.'

'Thank you, enjoy yoga.'

'Will do.'

'And Benji.'

'Sorry, what did you say?'

'Be bendy.'

'Right,' she replies.

There'll be butterflies in her tummy as she backs the car out of the drive. Stop being paranoid, she'll say to herself. Only she's right to be, because try as I might, sometimes I can't help myself.

When it's time, I head to the bottom of the garden to meet Morgan. I unlocked the gate the night after I gave her my phone which is how she must have discovered the fire escape that leads up to my balcony. She's in a hurry to leave, wants to take me somewhere.

'Put up your hood,' she says. 'Follow me.'

When we get to the end of the close, we cross over the road and enter the estate she lives on. We're immediately dwarfed by the buildings, a few people around but nobody bats an eye. Lights on in some of the windows, the late-afternoon sky darkening a little. Balconies stacked high with children's bikes, washing machines and junk.

'Hurry up, slow coach,' she says.

We walk to the tower block furthest into the estate, arrive at a set of stairs round the back.

'Where are we going?' I ask.

'All the way up,' and she points to the top of the building. 'Race you.'

She takes off first, but I soon catch her. Sixteen flights, no lights on the stairs, a door at the top, cobalt paint peeling off, the colour stands out from the grey concrete of the walls. We pause to catch our breath, smile at each other. She takes down her hood, I do the same.

'Come on,' she says.

She opens the door, the wind greets us with lust as we step out. Races up and over, crazy hard licks. She takes my sleeve, pulls me to the left. As we get closer to the edge of the roof I can see the world below. Cars and buses, people, no clue at all that we're up here watching them. She points to a part of the railing that's missing, says, be careful.

I nod. We walk towards a big air vent, a giant propeller encased in ribbed squares.

'Less windy here,' she says.

There's broken glass on the floor next to the vent, an empty Coke bottle. A plastic crate, two, maybe more. Cigarette butts scattered around. Ugly, yet beautiful, a place to be anonymous.

'Who comes up here?'

'Hardly anyone, just me usually. I don't live in this block but sometimes I come here to get away.'

I understand what she means, the need to get away sometimes. Often.

'How's the phone?' I ask her.

'All good, it was already unlocked so I got hold of a new SIM. Easy. Do you want it back?'

'No, I've got a new one, you hang on to it.'

'Are you sure?'

'Yeah. I've got something else as well.'

I take the wrap I stole from Saskia's purse out of my jeans pocket, hand it to her.

'No way, where did you get it?'

'Found it in my foster mum's handbag.'

'Jesus.'

I watch her unfold it crease by crease, until it lies open in her hand. She squats down, shields the contents, tells me she's had it a couple of times before at parties on the estate. She uses her pinkie to scoop some of the white powder on to her finger, leans in, plugs one nostril, sniffs the drug up the other. She passes the wrap to me, lies down immediately, a starfish on concrete. When she closes her eyes I pretend to inhale some. I fold it back up, lie down next to her.

'Fuck, that's good,' she says.

'Yeah.'

'So how's life with blondie?'

'I'm trying to stay out of her way.'

'Wise move, I don't reckon she's got a nice bone in her body.'

'Probably not.'

'So why were you sneaking around your foster mum's stuff anyway?'

'Just bored I guess, she's kind of easy to wind up as well.'

'So you like winding people up then?'

'Not really, I shouldn't do it to her. I reckon she's a bit scared of me.'

'Scared of you? As if. What's so scary about you?'

My past, is what's scary.

'Nothing. Here, have some more coke.'

Morgan's question unsettles me, makes me think about what lives inside me and if it's possible to outrun it. Traits buried deep in my DNA follow me. Haunt me.

She takes a line, jumps to her feet, asks me if I want to feel like I'm flying.

'Come on, I'll show you,' she says.

We walk to the edge of the roof, the gap in the barrier, the wind stronger, the sky darker. She's behind me, pushes me forward, close to the edge. Climb up, she says, on to the ledge. My body's rigid, my legs won't obey. It feels like a game I don't want to play.

'Go on, climb up, you won't fall. I do it all the time. Spread your arms out like an eagle.'

'No, it's too windy.'

She calls me a wimp, moves forward and steps on to the ledge, takes a moment to steady herself before uncurling her body from crouching, stands up.

One wrong move.

And.

Something switches on in my body.

'See,' she says, laughing. 'It's not hard, not for some of us anyway.'

Your voice comes to me now, it's angry, disappointed. SHE'S LAUGHING AT YOU, ANNIE, THAT'S NOT OKAY, FIND A WAY, MAKE HER PAY. No, I don't want to. I want to walk away but instead I take a step closer to her. A current runs up and down my spine, so dead since I left you, I don't know who I am. YES YOU DO, ANNIE, YOU DO KNOW, SHOW ME. I take another step, my arms stretch out so close to her, there on the edge, and maybe I would have, maybe I'm capable of it. Of worse. But she jumps down, turns to me, grinning, a chip in her front tooth. A powerful feeling of guilt when I look at her.

'Chicken,' she says. 'What do you want to do now?'

'I don't mind.'

'Let's go back to the air vent, take some more coke.'

'Okay.'

When we're lying on the ground again I ask Morgan why she wanted to fly, why she wanted to be like an eagle.

'To escape I suppose, go somewhere else.'

'Somebody once told me a story about a girl who was so scared she prayed to be given the wings of an eagle.'

'What was she scared of?'

The person who was telling her the story.

'Something was chasing her but no matter how fast she ran, or how far she went, it was always right behind her.'

'What was?'

'A serpent. It would wait until the girl was tired out from running, wait until she'd fallen asleep, and then it would come.'

'Is a serpent the same as a snake?'

'Yes.'

'Why was it after the girl?'

'It wasn't really a snake, it was just pretending to be one.'

'What was it then?'

'It was a person, letting the girl know if she ever tried to leave, it would come after her. Find her.'

'How can a person turn into a snake?'

'Sometimes people aren't what they say they are.'

'Does the girl get away?'

Not in the version you told me, Mummy.

'I don't know.'

'Why?'

'Because the girl disappeared and hasn't been seen since, and neither has the snake.'

'Do you think it's still chasing her?'

'Possibly.'

Probably.

'I'm glad no snakes are after me.'

'Yeah, lucky.'

'Have you got loads of other stories?'

'Yes.'

'Can you tell me another one?'

'Maybe next time.'

I got what I wanted, for Morgan and me to be friends, but now I'm afraid.

One wrong move.

And.

You mocked me in my head, said DON'T YOU SEE, ANNIE?

DON'T YOU SEE WHO YOU ARE?

11

When I get back to the house I see Mike's coat on the banister in the hallway, he must be home early from work. I collect my iPod from my room, not wanting to stay there alone, and head to the alcove outside his study. I like it there because it's an overspill for his books and a good spot, I've learnt, to listen in to his telephone conversations. The books in the alcove vary but mostly involve the study of all things 'psycho'. Psychoanalysis. Psychotherapy. Psychology. And a particular favourite of mine, a red hardback book on the study of psychopaths. The label given to you, by the press. Large and heavy the book is, a lot of chapters. Who knew they knew so much about you.

It's the chapter on the children of psychopaths that interests me the most. The confusion a child feels when violence is mixed with tenderness. Push and pull. A hyper vigilance, never knowing what to expect, but knowing to expect something. I recognize that feeling, I lived it every day with you. Like the time the power went off in our house, a storm outside. Worse inside. You got a torch, told me to go to the cellar, flick the circuit breaker back up. I told you I was scared, I didn't want to, I knew there was more than boxes and old furniture down there. You held the torch under your chin, told me you'd come with me, a trick, of course. You pushed me in, slid the bolt across. I clung to the door, counted backwards, a hundred or more, then I blacked out, woke up with you kicking me. You were disappointed in me, that's what you said, for being weak and afraid, vowed to toughen me up, teach me how to be just like you. That night I fantasized about turning the tables, ending your lessons, but I knew even if you were dead, your ghost would walk through walls until it found me.

I hear the phone in Mike's study ring, he answers quickly as if he expects it. I lift my headphones away from my ear, not that I have any music on, the trick, always look absorbed. Oblivious. Mike trusts me, no reason not to.

Yet.

A pause, then, hi, June, no problem at all, you're a good distraction for me, anything but write up today's notes. I know, tell me about it. Yes, she's fine, doing well at school, working hard. I'm trying to persuade Phoebe to do the same.

Laughter.

He doesn't speak for a while, listening to June, then says, god, poor girl, what more does she have to go through. I can't believe it.

A small explosion in my chest.

Mike goes quiet, listening again, then replies, yes, of course, I'll tell her about the trial-related stuff but not what her mum's saying. Thanks, June, I appreciate all the effort you're making. Yes, we think so too, very special indeed.

A click. Conversation over.

I replace my headphones, slide the red book under a cushion just before Mike comes out of the study. I pretend not to notice him, drum my fingers to the imaginary music I'm listening to. He waves his hand in front of me, I smile, press pause on my iPod, pull my headphones down.

'Hey, how was your day?' he asks.

'Okay thanks.'

'What are you reading?'

A heavy red book about Mummy. And me.

I hold up *Lord of the Flies*, the other book I'm reading.

'It's a set text. Miss Mehmet believes we should read at least one classic per month. It's also the play we're doing this term.'

'Did you get a part?'

'I missed the auditions but Miss Mehmet asked me to be the prompt, and I'm going to help out backstage, paint the scenery and stuff.'

'Nice. Did Phoebe get a part?'

Of course she did, she runs Year Eleven. Didn't you know?

'She's the onstage narrator, a lot of lines to learn.'

'Yikes, she'd better get busy then. Are you enjoying it?' He nods towards the book.

'Yeah, I am.'

'What do you like about it?'

'There's no adults.'

'Thanks,' he says, laughing.

'No, not like that.'

'Like what then? You like the fact the children don't have parents?'

'They do have parents, they're just not on the island with them.'

'Good point. But there's some pretty upsetting scenes though, aren't there?'

I nod, reply. 'Like Piggy's death.'

'Doesn't a boy called Simon die too?'

He noticed that I didn't mention that, the psychologist in him keen to explore why.

'Simon's death is very upsetting, don't you think?' he asks.

I hesitate for long enough to make it look like I'm giving it some thought, then reply.

'Yes.'

What I want to tell him. The truth. Is. I don't find the idea of people or children hurting and killing each other upsetting.

I find it familiar. I find it is home.

He sits down next to me. The sleeves of his shirt are rolled up, lightly coloured hair on his forearms, an expensive-looking watch. Close enough to touch me, but he won't.

'I've just been on the phone to June, she was checking in before she heads off for a few days of holiday.'

And reporting back to him whatever it is you're saying. Another plate on a pole, spinning.

'Is there any news about the trial? If I have to go or not?'

'Nothing concrete yet, but she did tell me the lawyers were putting together a series of questions for us to go through.'

'Questions?'

'Things you might be asked.'

'So I am going to be cross-examined then?'

'We're not sure yet and I know that's a horrible feeling, but I'll let you know as soon as I do. I promise.'

He stands up, stretches, offers to make me a snack, attempts to distract me. Stop me from asking any more questions. I walk through to the front part of the house with him.

'That reminds me, I forgot to tell you yesterday we're having a family dinner tonight.'

'All of us?'

'Yep. You, me, Sas and Phoebs.'

Pass the potatoes please, dog-face.

I wonder how that would go down at the table.

'We usually meet at about seven, is that okay?'

'Yeah.'

I spend the next couple of hours sketching and listening through the wall to Phoebe in her room, conversation after conversation on the phone. I think about knocking on her door, pretending it's the first time we've met.

Let's forget about everything that's happened so far, I'd say. Let's start again. Friends, even.

When it's time for dinner I go down to the kitchen, the smell of something roasting in the Aga, the air hot and uncomfortable. Mike feels it too, opens the window just after I arrive. Phoebe stands against the sink, head in her phone. There's a bottle of red wine open on the counter by the radio, which is off, nobody wants to run the risk of me hearing about you.

'Smells nice,' I say.

Phoebe looks up, scoffs, a dismissive noise from the base of her throat. Mike looks over at her, shakes his head. Saskia turns away, busies herself with stirring gravy on the stove top.

'That would be Sas's legendary roast chicken you can smell.'

'Legendary because it's so dry you'll be chewing until next Sunday. Not too late to order Chinese, peeps.'

Phoebe's comment is ignored, head drops down to her phone again. I'm new to this family but I feel it too. Saskia's inability to mother, to be strong. I look at Phoebe and it saddens me to think she can't see that she and I are more alike than we are not.

'Right, Phoebs, time to put the phone down, no arguments. Can you and Milly lay the table please.'

'Fine, just don't expect me to have fun.'

'Perhaps if you tried, you might,' Saskia says, turning to face us.

Her timing is off, years too late to soothe the angry ruffles of Phoebe's feathers. But why?

'Perhaps if I tried? Coming from you?'

'Please, guys, I don't think this is necessary in front of Milly.'

Wobbles, threatens to come toppling down. A deck of cards, carefully, painstakingly, arranged in a pyramid. Fragile family.

Nobody speaks, the only noise Rosie's paws on the tiles as she comes into the room, tail wagging, nose high in the air. A sneeze of pleasure as the scent of chicken now resting out of the oven tempts her, draws her near.

Mike leans down and scratches behind her ears, just where she likes it, then says, come on, old girl, out, and removes her, shuts her in the porch. Phoebe and I lay the table while Saskia serves up roast potatoes and veg into white bowls. When Mike comes back he sharpens a long knife, elaborate swishes and swipes, carves the chicken with it. He doesn't ask me to spread my fingers on the table while he stabs in between each one, as fast as he can. Not his kind of game.

Once we're seated it takes a few minutes of passing plates around, trading bowls from opposite sides of the table, for everybody to be ready to eat. Mike pours wine for Saskia and himself, and half a glass for Phoebe. When he offers me some, I say no, water is fine. Phoebe calls me a bore and we all laugh it off, I bet the name she calls me in her head is much worse.

'Cheers,' says Mike, raising his glass.

Nobody joins him.

'Milly tells me you're doing *Lord of the Flies* this term.'

He strikes gold, he knows where to mine.

'Yeah, I've pretty much got the biggest part, I'm onstage narrator. Miss Mehmet says it's because I've got such a clear voice.'

'That's nice to hear, isn't it, Sas?'

She nods, her heart's not in it though. Fantasizing about fucking Benji, or walking out the door, never coming back. Her eyes glassy, her hand reaching at her nose every now and then. Mike's not blind, nor blinkered. Chooses to ignore. Tolerate. Her stash, replenished. She's high. Fucked. Getting fucked. Fucking high.

'Milly. Earth to Milly,' I hear Mike say.

I'm staring again, this time at Saskia.

Phoebe makes the comment, if looks could kill. Saskia straightens up, attempts a mouthful of food. Mike says, enough now, that's enough. The conversation goes on. Bland. Tame. We eat while we talk. Phoebe was right though, the chicken's dry. Mike asks her how she's doing with learning her lines, suggests taking a leaf out of my book, reading and rereading the text. A red rag to a bull, a match to a flare.

'That's so typical, I've actually been working really hard on my lines, perhaps you're just too fucking busy to notice.'

She drains the wine in her glass, the heat of the alcohol adding fuel to her rage.

'Any more language like that and you'll leave the table, okay? Especially when your mum has cooked such a nice dinner.'

'I must be eating something else,' she replies.

Saskia's mouth opens, about to speak, but closes again, doesn't feel, and isn't, half as brave as her daughter. She excuses herself to the bathroom, her nose is hungry.

'It was only a joke, for god's sake.'

'Last warning, Phoebe, I mean it,' replies Mike.

She stabs her fork into a potato, looks at him, says, 'Fine.' He runs his hands through his hair, lets out a sigh, asks me if I'd like some more chicken.

'No thanks, I'm almost full.'

'Do I not get offered any?'

'Would you like some?'

'No, I'll have some more wine though.'

'Not tonight you won't.'

Too late. She picks up the bottle, half pours, half spills herself another glass. Full this time. Her lips, stained purple.

'I don't think so, Phoebe.'

He stands up, removes the glass from her hand, tips the wine down the sink.

'You never used to mind.'

'You used to behave better.'

She stares at me and I know somehow she's blaming me. When Mike sits back down he tries a different approach.

'Why don't you guys work together on the play, help each other out?'

'I'd like that,' I reply.

'Me and Iz are working on it together.'

'Perhaps you could include Milly?'

'She'd only be left out.'

'There's no need to be rude.'

'I'm not being rude, why are you taking her side?'

'I'm not taking anybody's side.'

'Yeah you are, I might as well be invisible.'

He could tell her, defuse the bomb. Explain why he and I spend so much time together, where we went when I missed school. The lawyers. Our evening conversations, what they're about. You. But he doesn't, he tells her it's important he helps me adjust to life as a member of the family, a little extra time and attention is needed. Phoebe's about to respond but Saskia comes back, heavy-bottomed glass in her hand. Ice. Slice of lime. She sits down, plays with her necklace, the gold one that matches Phoebe's, and mine. Phoebe doesn't miss a trick, not where her mother is concerned.

'Well, seeing as you've moved on to spirits, I might as well drink your wine.'

She reaches for Saskia's glass, drinks what's left of it. Lolita, a teenage temptress, knows all the buttons to push. Mike's hands press into the table, he'll be telling himself to calm down, employing tactics he uses in his work. He stands up, speaks.

'I'm not asking you, I'm telling you. Leave the table, Phoebe. If you're still hungry, take whatever you want with you, but go straight to your room and I'd prefer not to see you again this evening.'

She does as she's told. Steam runs low. What goes up, must come down.

And then there were three.

I can't help but feel sorry for her, I've felt it too. The hunger of loneliness around the people, or person, you're supposed to be protected by. Nurtured. Mike apologizes, asks me if I've had enough to eat.

'Yes thank you, I think I'll head up too if that's okay.'

'Of course, and I'm sorry, it wasn't supposed to be like this.'

I pause outside Phoebe's room, imagine what she's doing. Texting Izzy? Telling her how much she hates her family, how much she hates me?

No such thing as a shiny, new family.

'Milly, it's Mike, can you hear me?'

Please, stop crying.

'Milly, who are you talking to?'

I'm going to help you, I promise.

'Everything is okay, Milly.'

No, it's too late for that.

Somebody places their hands on my shoulders, holds them there. Applies pressure. A voice says, Milly, you need to come out of there. I open my eyes and I see Mike in front of me.

'Let me help you up.'

'No, they need me, Mike. They're frightened.'

'Take my hand, Milly. That's it, good girl.'

When Mike leads me out of the cellar, the light in the corridor blinds me. A spotlight. Exposed. This is who I am. I begin to cry, he holds me into his chest. His heart beats with something strong, I feel it through the thick material of his dressing gown. He's not supposed to touch me, but I'm glad he does.

'I'm sorry,' I say, deep into his chest.

'You have no reason to be sorry, Milly.'

I do.

I have many reasons.

12

Mike told me everything was okay when he took me back to my room on Saturday night, said we'd talk about it in this week's session, but how can I be sure he means it. That everything's okay. The ground beneath my feet, less firm when night comes. What I do, say. What I reveal about myself in those moments. My biggest fear was you, still is most of the time, but now I have a new fear, that I'll be shown the door, Mike recognizing he's bitten off more than he can chew. More than he wants to.

Eleven weeks today your trial begins. Eleven weeks, the same building as you, same air. I want to know what it was June told Mike on the phone. Something you've said. Something they don't want me to find out. Go slow and tell the truth, that's all you have to worry about, Mike said to me last week. Easy for him to say.

I sit up in bed, take one of the elastic bands from my wrist, pull my hair into a high ponytail, it's how the other girls wear it at school. Once I'm dressed I roll up the sketches I did over the weekend to show MK. I'm looking forward to seeing her again, I feel like I get it right when I'm with her. Just before I leave my room a text comes through. Morgan, saying she had fun on Saturday, see you soon, followed by a host of emojis. A star, a thumbs up. Two girls dancing in unison and a red balloon. She likes me, I think. Has seen only the good parts. Certain things should never be disclosed, that's what you used to say to me. Show only the side you know they'll like. Trust.

'Morning,' Mike says as I enter the kitchen.

'Morning.'

Phoebe is there, arms crossed over her chest, turns her face away when she sees me.

'Phoebe,' Mike says.

She looks up at him, exhales noisily and says, fine, then turns to me.

'Sorry about Saturday.'

I nod, reply.

'Thanks, it's okay.'

'No, it wasn't okay and she knows it. I've been very clear that if anything like that happens again, there'll be consequences. Right, Phoebe?'

'Yes.'

'Good,' Mike says. 'Now let's draw a line under this. Why don't you guys walk to school together? It's not often you leave at the same time.'

'I'm meeting Iz, we've got stuff to talk about.'

'As mentioned at dinner on Saturday, Phoebe, I'm sure you could include Milly from time to time. No?'

'It's okay, I like walking on my own, gives me a chance to clear my head.'

He looks disappointed, but lets it go. We finish breakfast at the same time and end up leaving together anyway, but when we exit the driveway, on to the main road, she says, 'Don't think I don't know what you're up to, but for the record, Mum and Dad never keep anyone longer than a couple of months. Pretty soon you'll be sent back to where you came from.'

She jogs away from me, rucksack bouncing, and joins

Izzy, who's waiting at the end of the road. Back to where you came from, she said. I want to shout after her, ask where does a person go if they can't stay where they are, or go back to the place they've come from. Where will I go after the court case is over? A temporary placement, that's what June said when I met her at the unit. Mike and Saskia have decided I'm the last foster child they'll take until Phoebe finishes her A levels. She has no idea how lucky she is and how much I wish there was room for us both.

When I get to school I check my timetable inside my locker. First period I'm supposed to have maths but as I walked past the office on the way in, there was a note pinned up outside announcing that Miss Dukes, our teacher, was off for the day, Year Elevens to work in the library. I decide to go to the art room first to see if MK is around. Her room is empty when I arrive, a tasselled cardigan hanging on the back of her chair, an art textbook open, face down on the desk. I want to turn it over, see what it is she's looking at, but the door to the corridor opens and she comes in carrying a pile of paper plates decorated with felt faces. She smiles when she sees me.

'This is a nice surprise. How was your weekend?'

'It was good, thank you. How was yours?'

'Pretty quiet, to be honest,' she replies. 'If it's me you're after you're in luck, I've got half an hour spare before the little ones pile in.'

'I wanted to show you some drawings I did over the weekend.'

'Wonderful, let's have a look then.'

I slide the roll of sketches out of my rucksack flap, hand them to her.

'Wow, you have been busy.'

'There's only three,' I reply, enjoying the way her enthusiasm makes me feel.

'Let's flatten them out on the table.'

We use pots of felt-tip pens to hold down the corners of the pages, she steps back when all three are laid out. Nods.

'These are great, particularly the girl with the eagle wings. Have you always liked to draw?'

'I think so, yes.'

'Are either of your parents artistic?'

How to tell her, how to explain that you believed what you did was art.

Skin, not paper.

'My mum left when I was young, so I'm not really sure.'

'Sorry, that was insensitive of me to ask, I know you're staying with the Newmonts.'

I tell her it's fine, but it's not. It's not what she said, it's what I can't.

'You're very talented. Have you thought about studying art once you finish school?'

'Maybe, but I also really like science.'

'Better money in science, that's for sure. Thanks for sharing them with me, I love to see what you girls come up with. If you don't mind I have to reply to some emails but feel free to stay and do some drawing for the next twenty minutes or so.'

'I'm supposed to be in the library. Miss Dukes is off so we've got a study period instead.'

'I can give the librarian a quick call if you like, let her know you're with me.'

'You don't mind me staying?'

'Of course not, the more the merrier. It's nice to have company, isn't it?'

Yes.

I sit at one of the easels while she phones Mrs Hartley, reach for a red piece of chalk from the box on the table next to me. I sweep, swirl. We work in silence. Dust flies, so does time. Red splinters stand out against the navy of my school skirt. I press too hard, the chalk breaks.

'May I see?' she asks.

'Yeah.'

She walks over, stands behind me.

'The colour in this piece is very powerful.'

I nod.

The spillages and seepages.

'Can you describe what you've drawn? Is that a person there?'

MK's finger hovers close to your face, but doesn't touch it. She traces the air around it, does the same for the red sweeps of chalk surrounding you.

'It's an interpretation of something I saw.'

'Something on TV?'

'Something like that, yes.'

'Have you heard of the Sula Norman Art Prize?'

'Is that the girl who died?'

'Yes, she died of leukaemia two years ago. A very talented artist I believe, although I never met her, before my time here. When she passed away her parents pledged an art prize to the school, a year's supply of art materials and an exhibition at a gallery in Soho. Having seen your work, I'd recommend you enter it.'

'I'm not sure I'm good enough.'

'Trust me, if you keep turning out work like this I think you've got a strong chance of winning. I shouldn't say that, but it's true.'

'Thank you, I'll think about it.'

I walk to the sink, focus on washing my hands, anything but the warmth spreading across my face. Stupid to blush, and she noticed. I pull a paper towel from the dispenser, dry my hands. She joins me at the sink, gives me a damp cloth.

'For the dust on your skirt,' she says.

I spend the remainder of the period in the library, and leave as fast as possible when the bell goes, make sure I get to the gym before the others. I change in a cubicle. Private. My body's my own these days, leotard on for vaulting practice. I'm glad I didn't cut last night, Mrs Havel's arms support either side of my ribs as she helps us turn headfirst over the vaulting horse. A younger pupil comes in and interrupts the lesson.

'There's an important phone call for you, Mrs Havel.'

'Can't it wait?'

'No, Mrs McD in the office said it was urgent.'

'Okay, I won't be a minute, girls. Lay off the vaulting and do some mat work instead and for goodness' sake no messing about, be careful.'

The noise rises as soon as the door to the gym closes. Laughter and teasing, conversations about boys and things that happened over the weekend. I listen, it helps me learn how to fit in. Blend in. I watch Georgie, one of the smallest girls in the year, climb up a rope attached to the ceiling. She uses her feet to push against the large knot at the bottom, her arms to pull up, gain height. She's doing well, almost halfway, the rope swings a little from side to side as she continues. I see Phoebe nudge Clondine, whisper something, then giggle and approach the rope. Georgie's high up now, no crash mat, I know what they're about to do, I can tell. I should intervene but for once it's not me being ridiculed. Belittled.

They start to swing the rope, gently at first. It doesn't take long for the other girls to notice. The crowd soon gathers, high ponytails dip down as necks bend and heads look up to the roof. Phones would be too, but no pockets in the leotards. Georgie tells them to stop, but they don't. Climb down, quick, I want to yell, but fear gets to her first. Tells her to hang on, whispers in her ear, hang on for your life. She pulls her body in close, tightens her grip round the rope, bare feet useless. Slips a little, scrambles up. One leg released, clamped in again. Somebody makes a joke, says what's the weather like up there, Georgie. Laughter. Swearing. Oh fuck, look how high she's swinging. Then a warning from Annabel.

'She's going to fall, Phoebe, stop it.'

But she doesn't listen, she pulls harder on the rope, her smile bigger, enjoying the power. The control. Georgie swings like a baby monkey without its mother's back or tail to hang on to. No branches, no trees. Nothing to break the fall. Up there alone. Out there alone. We all are.

'Go on, Clon, your turn.'

She does as she's told, pulls the rope to the left, spins Georgie around. Every time the rope turns I can see her eyes, wet. Tears. Frightened. Body slips a little, more than last time. Tired. Help her. Can't. Can. Don't want to.

Nobody helped me.

The rope begins to slow, Clondine steps away, calls to Georgie.

'That'll be a tenner for the ride, please.'

The other girls lose interest, they presume only a good outcome, that the rope will no longer be swung, that Georgie will slide down to the ground in a minute or so, complaining to Phoebe and Clondine about how scared she was. The circle of spectators begins to disintegrate into twos and threes, wander away. The rope, almost stationary now. A cartwheel competition begins on the mats, gossiping resumes. Most of the girls, but not Phoebe. Whatever it is, it lurks in her too, she can't resist one last pull on the rope. A fire inside her burning just that little too brightly.

Georgie, too tired to hang on.

I look away before she hits the ground. The noise, distinctive. Bones do that. Pop. Crack. The laughter I joined in with minutes ago peters off to silence. Silence becomes fuck.

'You fucking idiot, Phoebe,' Clondine says.

I turn round. Georgie. More slumped than sitting, face white, the same colour as the bone jutting out from under her chin. A knife of calcium, a collarbone. A flurry of leotards, no longer cartwheeling, move, flock around her. I move too, but round the back, sit down next to her. Breath, hers, coming in short gasps, the rope swinging accusingly over our heads. We all had a part to play. The noise in the gym different now, pitches higher than before, a panicky edge. The girls cling to each other, trauma.

'Fuck. It wasn't just me, it was you as well, Clondine.'

'No, I'd walked away at that point and so should've you.'

'Oh my god, I think I'm going to be sick.'

'Shut up, Clara, think about poor Georgie.'

'We'll get you to Jonesy, okay, Georgie? You're going to be okay,' says Annabel. Decisive. Captain-like.

Phoebe squats down, she has a small window of opportunity to make this right and she knows it. She's straight in there.

'I'm so sorry, I thought you were on your way down. I would never have done it if I thought you were going to fall.'

'It's a little bit late for that, don't you think?' Annabel responds.

'Would you shut the fuck up for once, go and get Jonesy and bring her here and don't you dare say anything. Anyway, everybody will back me up, right? We were all laughing, we're all to blame, it was an accident.'

She's good. So very good. The girls nod in solemn agreement. Clara turns away and gags into her hand, shoulders heaving. Georgie begins to moan. An eerie sound that grows into a wail when she looks down, sees the bone piercing her skin. Annabel sprints to the door, shouting behind her, I'm getting Jonesy.

'Don't look,' I tell Georgie.

Phoebe hears Georgie's wailing the loudest, wants it to stop.

'Fuck,' she says. 'Calm down, please, Jonesy will be here soon. Just remember to say it was an accident, okay?'

'Shall I get her some water?' asks Marie.

'No,' somebody replies. 'You shouldn't give her anything to drink, I saw it on the telly, just keep her warm until help gets here.'

'What about the hoodie over there, should we put it over her legs? Are you cold, Georgie?'

I feel her body begin to shake. Shock. I lean her back into my shoulder.

'Why don't we try and get her up, sit her on the

bench?' suggests Phoebe. 'Can you do that, Georgie, can you manage?'

She shakes her head, begins to cry.

'You have to try, come on, let's help her up.'

I know what Phoebe's trying to do, to 'clean up' the scene, make it look less savage. The broken body of a girl looks better on a bench than it does slumped under the rope she fell from, was spun from.

'No, don't,' I hear myself say.

A sea of purple and blue velour stares at me.

'Mind your own business,' Phoebe replies.

'She's in too much pain, you can't move her.'

'And what makes you such an expert on broken bones?'

A movement on my scalp, a slow creeping heat. I support Georgie's weight, tell her to hold her elbow, cradle her arm into her stomach.

'Yes, like that, it'll help with the pain.'

It helped with mine.

Jonesy, the school nurse, arrives, takes one look at Georgie and tells Annabel to go to the office and call an ambulance. She pushes a vault in behind us, thanks me for helping and tells Georgie to lean back gently. Mrs Havel must have heard the news too, arrives looking furious.

'What happened?' she asks. 'I told you to be careful.'

'We were,' replies Phoebe. 'We were just having a bit of fun and then Georgie fell from the rope.'

'Were none of you listening? I said mat work only. Go and get changed, all of you, hurry up.'

Phoebe's waiting for me outside my cubicle, comes up to my face, so close I see tiny brown flecks bedded into the blue of her eyes.

'Next time, don't get involved in things that don't concern you, okay?'

I ignore her, walk away. She follows, shoves me backwards as she passes. I land hard on the wooden changing benches.

Bruised, but alive.

So very alive, Phoebe.

13

A few days after the gym incident, Phoebe passes round a
card at the end of biology.

'Everybody sign it,' she orders. 'I'll get Mrs McD to send
it home to Georgie.'

When the card gets to me, I read Phoebe's pink swirls —
Sorry about your accident, get better soon, love P xxx.

'Your accident', an interesting choice of words. Reads nice,
to a teacher or parent. No reason to suspect foul play, and
Georgie knows better than to squeal. Everybody does, but
me, I squealed on you, didn't I, Mummy? I told the story
again and again, a blinking red light from the video camera.

When everybody's signed it I watch Phoebe lick the flap,
press it down with one hand, a smooth V-shaped motion.
She applies Vaseline to her lips, the colour pink, kisses the
centre of the V on the back of the envelope. I think about
how different she is at school. So self-assured. How different I was as well, so good at pretending, at keeping our
secrets. I wonder what the girls would think if they knew
that Phoebe calls out in her sleep. Cries. I've heard her on
the nights I'm too frightened to sleep, too frightened to
stay in my room, all the shadows and whispering from
dark corners. From you. Sometimes I get up, sit in the corridor nestled into the long velvet drapes. Restless and
troubled Phoebe is, small lonely yelps in her sleep that turn
into tears when she wakes up. Sometimes a lamp goes on, a
slice of bright underneath the door. I've thought about

going in, telling her it's okay, though likely it's not. I'm not sure which is worse, a mother like mine that was too much, or one like Phoebe's. Not enough.

The bell goes for lunch and I head over to the prep school. I've only helped out twice before but the kids seem to like me and I like them. I find their company to be a little like magic. They exist half in our world, half in theirs. Dragons to be slayed, princesses to rescue. Read it again, Milly, we love this story, pl-e-e-e-e-e-ease. One of the girls fell over last week, I rubbed her hands, brushed the gravel from her knees. Be brave, I told her, you'll need to be.

When I arrive in the playground a small crowd runs at me, smiles and arms outstretched. 'Yay, Milly's here.'

'Can we play horsey?' asks Evelina, a tiny fragile-looking girl, pale skin, pink around her eyes. A mummy at home, who I bet runs oatmeal baths for the dry patches of eczema, visible behind her knees.

'Climb on then,' I reply, bending so she can reach.

I do it a lot. Think about what sort of parents other children have. The staff at the unit were so quick to tell me what you did was wrong. Abnormal. So I'm trying to learn what's right, I'm trying to be different from you.

Evelina, a koala, locks her arms round my neck. As we canter past a classroom window, a trail of kids running behind, keen for it to be their turn next, I catch a glimpse of my reflection. I look away.

When I bend down, let Evelina slide off, a chorus of 'me next' starts up. I make a big show of pretending to look overwhelmed, run in a circle, they follow, of course. One girl lags behind, eyes trained on the floor, occasional glances, watches the other children, how they interact with me. I remember doing the same when I was her age. I offer her my back to climb on.

'Would you like a go?' I ask.

She shakes her head, fiddles with the buttons on her blazer, looks away. A chubby girl I'm keen to avoid launches herself at my back, tells me to giddy up. I'm angry that the other little girl, the one I want, doesn't trust me enough to join in. You taught me how to be with children, yet it seems I still lack a lot of your charm. Your skill.

I take off, galloping.

'Faster, faster,' demands the shrill voice behind me.

She squeezes her legs round my waist, the sensation bothers me. Suffocates me. It's a big drop from my back, not as far as Georgie's fall but enough to hurt a five- or six-year-old. I should hold her tight.

I should.

She lands with a thump, begins to cry.

'You dropped me.'

'Oh, come on, Angela, no need for dramatics. All good riders take a tumble every now and then. Pick yourself up, dust yourself down.'

And move along. Out of my sight.

Hopscotch squares are painted on to some of the concrete slabs of the playground. I see the little girl pretending to look down at them. I don't ask her to play, I know she won't, but I walk over, give her a sweet from my pocket. Children like sweets, and the people who give them to them.

Your praise follows immediately – THAT'S MY GIRL – but instead of leaving me feeling victorious as it did in the toilets with Clondine and Izzy, this time it leaves me feeling sordid.

'Hey, not fair,' says Angela, when she notices the sweet. 'I was the one that fell.'

I ignore her. Fat. Little. Piggy. The bell rings, signals the end of lunch.

'Come on, everyone, let's form a train and choo-choo to the registration point.'

Three teachers wait to sign the children back in, a head-count each time. You never know who lurks outside the playground.

Or in it.

'Miss Carter, Milly dropped me.'

'What's that, Angela?'

I answer instead.

'It was just a game, we were playing horsies, all okay though.'

'Hmm, well please be more careful next time, Milly, the last thing we need is a complaint from a parent.'

'Sure, I'll be careful.'

'Do,' she replies, beady eyes on me.

I meet her stare, smile. It's not me who should be careful.

Miss Evans, one of the other teachers, asks the kids to thank me. They do it in unison, a beautiful birdsong. It fills me, warms me. I look for the girl. She's at the back of the line, still trying to look small. Invisible.

Mike came home late from work yesterday so we only managed a short session. He wanted to talk to me about Daniel, about the possibility of what I'd be asked if I'm cross-examined in court, how the defence might try to imply I should have done more. Could have done more. It's vital you resist internalizing these feelings, he said, hang on to the reality that none of it was your fault. Nobody blames you. *Not true*, I wanted to say.

I blame me.

He asked to meet again tonight so we could continue with guided relaxation, said it's crucial for releasing trauma buried in my subconscious. I told him I don't like not being able to remember everything I've said. You have to trust me, Milly, he replied, I know what I'm doing, I've been doing it for a long time.

Before I meet with him I reply to Morgan's text from earlier. She said she'd been spying on the 'blonde bitch' and did I know she smoked? No I didn't, I reply. I see her writing a response – Well she does, wonder what else I can find out about her?!! I never asked her to, but I like the idea of her creeping about, spying for me, it makes me feel closer to her, like she's someone I can trust.

When I arrive in the kitchen Phoebe's telling Mike about Georgie's accident and how she helped. She goes on to tell him I froze, didn't help at all. As pale as Georgie was.

'Never mind,' he says, looking at me. 'Sounds like it was good you were there, Phoebs.'

'Also, Dad, have you seen a chemistry paper of mine lying around?'

'I don't think so, darling. When did you last have it?'

'I'm not sure, yesterday maybe, but it's due for tomorrow and Mr Frith will flip out if I don't hand it in.'

'You better get searching then.'

Saskia joins us, dressed in yoga gear. Vagina obvious as ever.

'Did you hear that, Sas? Phoebs helped Georgie Lombard, she had an accident in the gym a few days ago.'

'That's nice,' she replies. 'I have to shoot though, I'm late for class.'

It stings Phoebe. The fact she doesn't ask for more details. She gives Saskia a filthy look and pushes past her. Saskia gestures to Mike and says, what?

'Nothing,' he replies. 'Come on, Milly, we should get started.'

None of us notice her at first. Three. Floors. Up. Perched on the edge of the banister.

'Enjoy yoga, Mummy dearest,' she says, looking down at us.

She taunts Saskia, takes her hands off the banister, does a faux wobble, wants her to say be careful, but it's not her, it's Mike who says it.

'Don't be so stupid, come down from there, it'll be the death of you.'

Let down again, she flicks her middle finger at her mum, disappears off the landing into her room. Mike attempts a smile, but Saskia replies with: 'You're the psychologist, fix it.'

'Sas, she's our daughter, not something to fix. She's angry because –'

'Because of me, that's what you were going to say, wasn't it?' Saskia replies. 'It's my fault. It was years ago now but it's still my fault, right?'

'That's not what I meant. Look, I'll talk to her, just not tonight.'

'Perhaps if you spent more time with your own daughter things would improve.'

A low blow, she's sorry as soon as she says it, apologizes immediately. I stare at her thin body, not much different in size from Phoebe's, same hair, eyes. Much like a teenager herself but out of her depth in a house with us teenage-for-real girls. The lessons these days, faster. Cruder.

On the way to Mike's study he explains that the psychiatrist from the unit called him today, checking in about my current medication regime. I remember his office well. Walls full of framed degrees and certificates. The questions, the same every week. Appetite. Headaches. Flashbacks. And finally, sleep. How are you sleeping? Every night's different, I told him. Yes, to be expected, he replied. A rip of a pad, another cocktail of pills ordered. Blue for the morning, white for the night. Pink, if I didn't want to think at all. One of the other teenagers showed me how to hold them in the side of my mouth, spit them out in the toilet afterwards.

Taking them felt like cheating.

A kindness I didn't deserve, still don't when I think back to what I let happen to Daniel the night before I handed you in.

'How would you feel about increasing your night-time dose?' Mike asks.

I tell him I feel groggy at school, first thing in the morning.

'Still? That's not great, let me note that down so I remember to mention it when I call him back tomorrow. We'll arrange a full review once the trial's over.'

Mike, so diligent at dispensing my medication. Not so at making sure I take them. A sock full of tablets in my top drawer. He opens his diary, writes a note in it, then sits down in the chair opposite me.

'Ready?' he asks.

'Not really.'

'This is important work, Milly. There are parts of your mind we need to access in order for you to be able to move on. For example, the night-time episode you had a few days ago in the cellar when you were dissociating is linked to guilt, and how you feel about the things you did that weren't your fault.'

Fear inches up from the lower part of my stomach, moves into my throat.

'You need to address these feelings, you need to feel secure in the fact your mother can't control you any more.'

Mike said yesterday he knew what he was doing, he'd been doing it for a long time, so why can't he see the strings, yours, attached to me still? Why can't he see what's going on?

'Let's do some relaxing and we can talk more at the end.'

He makes me visualize my safe place but all I can see are faces of ghosts, forming in smoke. The cigarette you enjoyed afterwards. The little ghosts swooping still. They can't rest in peace, they don't like where they are.

Where they were put.

'Describe what you can hear,' Mike asks.

'Somebody calling for help.'

'Who is it?'

'Somebody in the room opposite mine.'

'Did you go and look, see who it was?'

'I knew who it was, I recognized his voice, but the door was locked, I couldn't get to him.'

'It wasn't your job to help him, Milly.'

'The next morning he was crying, asking for his mummy, but the door was still locked so I couldn't help him then either. Then we left the house and she drove me to school, sang the same song every time.'

'What song did she sing?'

'Lavender's green, dilly dilly, lavender's blue.'

IF YOU LOVE ME, DILLY DILLY, I WILL LOVE YOU. YOU STILL LOVE ME, DON'T YOU, ANNIE?

'I was there too, Mike.'

'Where were you, Milly?'

I open my eyes. He's leaning forward in his chair.

'You said you were there too, what did you mean?'

I bite down on my tongue. Bitter and warm as the blood flows.

'You did everything you could, Milly. Everything you could in the circumstances. It must be especially hard remembering Daniel.'

'Why do you think it was him I was remembering?'

'You recognized his voice. He was the only one you knew well enough.'

'But that doesn't mean I didn't care about all of the children she took.'

'I know, and I'm not saying you didn't, but it must have been that much harder when you realized it was Daniel she'd taken, you'd spent time with him at the refuge.'

'I don't want to talk about it.'

'But you need to. You need to be able to if you go to court.'

'I will be able to by then.'

'Why not try now?'

'I feel like you're pressuring me, I need more time.'

'I just want you to know this is a safe space, Milly, you can tell me anything, talk to me. That's what I'm here for.'

I tell him I know, but I'm tired, and I don't want to talk any more.

He sits back in his chair, nods, says, okay, let's leave it there for tonight.

I read until midnight, exhausted, yet sleep doesn't come. I long to be held, comforted by someone. How your touch hurt, how no touch hurts more. I get out of bed, unlock the balcony door, open it wide. Cold air floods the room, every shiver and goosebump on my body a welcome sensation. My lonely skin.

I sit down on the stool in front of the easel Mike and Saskia bought me. Kindness from them, every day. It's late now, past two a.m. The night air wraps around me, my feet hum from exposure. I like the noise charcoal makes. The smudges, the smears, perfection left out in the cold. The black on my hands reminds me something is happening. Being done. I rock on the stool as I sketch, back and forward. I close my eyes for a moment, my grip on the charcoal tightens. The wind reaches through the balcony door, pinches my breasts. My nipples, hard and tight.

I rock to the side.

The left and the right. A circular motion. I enjoy the wood of the stool through my knickers, the heat created, a stark contrast to the rest of my cold body. I rub.

Harder on the page.

Harder on the stool.

The charcoal breaks. I'm left with a pulse down below, black dust on my knees.

In the morning a sketch clipped to the easel. You, again. I remove the paper, roll it up, place it in the pull-out drawer under my bed.

14

The past few days haven't been good. A recurring dream about being on the stand, opening my mouth, but instead of words, a colony of bats flies out. Screeching the truth. The shame of saying it out loud, of what I let you do to me. Of what I let you do to them. I woke up this morning gasping for breath, the pillow game you used to play.

Morgan didn't reply to my messages over the weekend. She sometimes helps her uncle out so I know that'll be what it is but I've often wondered what would happen if she found out about me. Whether she'd understand, still want to be my friend. I've thought about telling her. She's the person I feel closest to, and sometimes the burden of you is too much on my own. The need to share, to feel normal. I'm not sure if she'd keep it secret though and I worry that if the parents of the children you took can't get to you, they might come after me. A child for a child.

I choose a black hoodie and jeans. Uggs. Today we're going on a school trip with Brookmere College, and I've been dreading it since it was announced. Visible I feel, for all the wrong reasons, the other girls, confident. Know how to act around boys. In the kitchen there's a note from Mike, along with a plate of croissants: 'Monday treat, enjoy the trip, girls.'

The way he pluralizes me and Phoebe. A team. I wouldn't mind it being true, we'd make a good one. Saskia comes in, asks if I'm looking forward to the trip.

'Sort of.'

'Better than lessons, surely?'

Not really, no.

'Here, take a croissant with you.'

'Thanks. Has Phoebe left already?'

'About five minutes ago, I think.'

'Okay, see you later.'

I chuck the croissant in the bin on the way to school, stomach all over the place. I'm hoping to see MK this afternoon when we get back, show her more of my work. She nods and smiles whenever she sees me at school. Last Friday she stopped at my table during lunch, wished me a nice weekend. I found myself imagining what my life would've been like if I'd grown up with her instead of you. I felt guilty afterwards, almost immediately.

The bus is outside school when I arrive, registration on board. Hurry up, everyone, on you go, says Mr Collier, one of the classics teachers. I choose a seat near the front, less likely anybody will sit next to me. Headphones on, no music though. The bus fills quickly, energy full and ripe. The girls aglow, an extra layer of bronzer applied, perfume sprayed liberally. The boys, like apes, do pull-ups on the overhead luggage rack. A zoo. Overwhelming. A headcount is done, somebody shouts from the back, Joe's missing, a joke about him taking a dump. Limits are set by Mr Dugan, the boys' teacher.

'I see him, sir, he's coming.'

'Hurry up, Joe. No, you can't, we've waited long enough for you, just sit in the first seat you find, please.'

He looks towards the back, shrugs, drops into the seat next to me. Catcalls and whistles follow, he holds his middle finger up in the air.

'Pipe down, the lot of you,' Mr Dugan says, through the microphone. 'We should get there in about forty minutes or so, traffic dependent. When we arrive you are not to wander off, understood? Disembark from the bus, go inside and wait as a group at the ticket desk. Please remember, all of you, even out of uniform you represent both schools. Any questions?'

'Can we stop at McDonald's?'

'Any sensible questions? No. Excellent. Sit back and enjoy the view and for goodness' sake, Oscar Feltham, take your feet off the seats, manners of a pig.'

I can see Joe looking at me, little sidelong glances, checking for my second head. I turn further towards the window, away from him, yet the smell of him follows. A spicy depth, some kind of spray deodorant, not unpleasant though the thought embarrasses me. He asks me something. My instinct is to ignore but he says it again, leaning forward in his seat so he's in my line of vision. I lift one of my headphones away from my ear, turn to face him. Hair, ginger. Eyes, blue.

'Sorry, what was that?'

'Would you like some chewing gum?'

'No thanks.'

'Oh go on, it's the menthol one, dead strong.'

He holds the packet towards me. No thanks, I tell him again, wishing I was able to relax, act in a more normal, open way. More practice needed. He withdraws his hand, shrugs, puts a piece in his mouth, letting out an exaggerated breath moments later as the menthol kicks in. He smiles and says, probably should have said no as well, opens his mouth, pants a little. I don't want to see his tongue, so I look away.

'Have you been to the London Dungeon before?' he asks.

Somewhere very similar.

'No.'

His voice is low, he doesn't want the back of the bus to know we're talking.

'Neither have I, should be a real laugh though.'

I don't reply, I don't agree.

'You don't look that keen.'

'Not really.'

'How come?'

'I'm not feeling very well.'

'You're not going to spew, are you?' He smiles as he says it.

'I don't think so, no.'

'Phew. You're not from here, are you? I know you're staying with Phoebe and her folks for a bit.'

I nod.

'Whereabouts are you from?'

'I've moved around a lot.'

'That's cool, I've only ever lived here. I'm Joe by the way.'

'Milly.'

'So how is life in the Newmont household?'

'It's okay.'

'Phoebe not being a pain in the arse then?'

The surprise on my face lasts long enough for him to notice. He winks at me. Oh god.

'Come on, I've known her for years, she can be a real bitch. Pretty hot, but still a bitch.'

'She's not all bad.'

'Really? That surprises me, she's not one for competition.'

'I'm not in competition with her.'

'She'll see it that way, trust me, and because you're different she won't be a happy bunny.'

I can't bring myself to ask him what he means by different. The suspicion of a set-up between Phoebe and him, a conversation late at night where she asked him to pretend to like me, then make me look like a fool.

'Being different is good by the way. Trust me, I'm ginger.'

He smiles again, then asks, 'Are you coming to Matty's party at half-term?'

Another hot topic on the forum. Free house, carnage. Teenagers' default mechanism is. Party. I'm not sure I got that gene.

'I haven't been invited.'

'I'm inviting you.'

'I'm not really into parties.'

'Everyone's going, it'll be a real laugh. You and Phoebs should come together, Matty's house is only a few streets from yours.'

'Not sure, maybe. I might listen to my music now if that's okay.'

'Sweet, I'll catch a few zeds before we get there.'

I feel relieved when it's over. The conversation. And when the bus pulls up outside the Dungeon we pile off, and Joe rejoins his group. The girls stay close to the boys, or the boy they laid dibs on weeks ago. What happens less than twenty minutes later is my fault. I let my guard down after talking to Joe. Kindness is lethal.

The front of the group is where I'd planned to be, close to the teachers and tour guide with his blood-stained costume and brown teeth, but I've ended up nearer the back. Phoebe and her gang are there and Claudia, the German exchange student, more interested in kissing the boy she's with than the displays. Phoebe calls her a slag, pushes past her. The lighting in the tunnel is low, throwing shadows small and large up the walls. Every now and then screams are released from speakers hidden somewhere, and laughter. Nasty laughter, a torturer enjoying his job. A head being chopped off. A sensation of being followed. Watched. Eyes hidden in the dark, the skin on my scalp pulls tight. Gunshot flashes of a place I've been to that looks like this, a place I never want to go to again.

I try to focus on the sounds around me, I try not to listen to your voice. Goading me. YOU WERE THERE TOO, ANNIE. I watch how the boys take pleasure in pretending to trip up the girls. Grab them. Grope them. The girls giggle and push them away, only to return to their sides moments later. More screams released, rats running overhead. A toothless woman begging, a dead baby by her side, a crow pecking at its eye. You say it again. YOU WERE THERE TOO, ANNIE.

Eyes like pools. Threaten to overflow. Tears. Hot. I push my way through the group, try to get to the front, find some air. Light. I don't even notice I'm not the one pushing any more. Phoebe is, and a few other hands too. They push me into one of the prison cells, barricade the door, and I know there's no point in shouting.

Help.

Numbers make me feel safe but not when I know approximately sixty pupils separate me from the teachers and the exit. I try to remember my breathing exercises, the panic attacks I experienced in the first couple of weeks after I left you. In through my mouth, out through — No, the other way, in through my nose, out through my mouth.

Pitch black.

I try the cell door again, but somebody's holding it shut. I sense a movement behind me. Three small lights embedded in the floor switch on, highlight a shadow. A display, not real.

It's okay, I can do this.

A figure by the wall, a woman. I press the back of my hand into my mouth, I don't want to scream. Tears prick at my eyelids. Memories pinch and grab me, like fish feeding on bread in a pond. HELLO, ANNIE. No, go away, you're not real. TURN ROUND, ANNIE. No. I lean into the door, close my eyes, bang my fists on the metal.

'Let me out, please, let me out.'

I hammer on the door. Head swimming. Images of me, carrying something in my arms, opening a door. Dark, so dark. The smell. Rotten, yet sweet. A low hum of activity, flies hatching. Rats scratching.

I didn't want to. I didn't.

You. Made. Me.

NOT ALWAYS, ANNIE.

That's not true.

I see their faces, the faces I try so hard not to see, small and afraid. Can't get to them. Crying. I close my eyes. Shout.

'Let me out, please. Somebody let me out.'

Please.

I feel hands on me.

'You're okay, chill out, you're fine. Open your eyes.'

Laughter as I do. I'm hunched in the corner of the cell, my arms round my head, covering my ears.

'Hurry up, Mr Collier's calling us,' says a girl's voice.

Joe's there, he offers me his hand. I refuse, not sure if he was in on it.

'Are you okay? You seem really freaked out.'

'That's because she is a freak,' says Phoebe.

'Shut the fuck up, can't you see she's terrified?'

'Oooooh, someone's got a crush on dog-face.'

'Dog-face? Have you looked in the mirror recently?'

'Nice try, Joe, we all know that's not what you were saying at Lucille's party.'

'Yeah well, I'm not wasted now, am I?'

'Must be if you're trying to help her.'

'Sound a bit jealous if you ask me.'

'Jealous? Of her?' As I stand up, she points at me.

'Looks that way, yeah.'

'Fuck off, Joe.'

She shoves him in my direction, heads up the passage towards the next exhibit. I hear Mr Dugan telling us to hurry up, another group's due behind us. My left nostril feels warm and full. Stress, anxiety, any kind of heightened emotion, triggers it. I tell Joe to leave me alone, turn my face away.

'Let's walk up together,' he says.

'No, please go away.'

He hesitates, but walks off, just before my nose begins to bleed.

We return to school in time for lunch and spend the rest of the afternoon setting up the Great Hall for Subject Evening, a chance for parents to come in and discuss career choices for their daughters. General feedback on how we've settled into the first few weeks of term. Mike and Saskia attend and ask to speak to both Phoebe and me when they get home. Phoebe goes first, I wait in the snug. After a while she comes out of the kitchen, slams the door behind her, gives me a hateful look as she passes.

Mike opens the door, I ask him if Phoebe's okay. He explains she got a double detention for losing her chemistry paper. Shame, I think, I could have told her where it was, the drawer under my bed. A small price to pay for Georgie's 'accident'.

Mike does most of the talking. Reports that I'm amongst the top five academically in Year Eleven, a little unsure in the social aspect, but making progress. Saskia squeezes my shoulder, it doesn't make me feel good, it makes me think of you. Parents' evening last summer, I was there helping. You wore a dress, red and blue flowers. One of the teachers commented on how well-mannered and compliant I was, wanted to know what your secret was. You squeezed my shoulder, replied with a smile, don't know, lucky I guess.

'Miss Kemp told us she encouraged you to enter the art prize.'

'I didn't really want to but she thinks I've got a good chance of winning. I'm working on some sketches for it.'

'Sounds like you and she are a great match,' Mike says.

'I really like her.'

And as I say it out loud, I realize it's true.

When I check my phone later, Morgan's replied.

Sorry for not being in touch my little shit of a brother hid my phone, can't see you this week but let's do something over the weekend. Something fun

You used to say the same thing on the drive back from school on a Friday afternoon. Something fun. One time I thought about jumping out of the car when it was moving, but somehow you knew. Flicked the child locks on. Big mistake, Annie, you said. I thought you would own less of me after I handed you in but sometimes it feels you own more. Something as innocent as a school trip becomes a walk down memory lane with you. Invisible chains. Jangle when I walk.

Up eight. Up another four.
The door on the right.

This time, a girl.
Not your first choice, only took them if you had to.
Two of the nine.
Asked me if I was watching.
I was. The bravest, and saddest I saw.
She kept getting up, after each blow.
I wept into the peephole, made sure I'd stopped crying before
you opened the door.
I wrapped her up, a coal sack, blankets forbidden for girls.
I carried her down, placed a doll next to her, used to be mine.
Her body, so still.
Shh little one, it's over now.

A couple of days ago Mike and I met as usual for our Wednesday session. I told him the truth, that I was frightened, that during the day I hear you, your voice in my head. I wanted to tell him about the nights too, you as a ribbon of dread lying next to me in bed, but I was ashamed. He asked me what it is you say to me. I told him you say I'm useless, that I won't manage life without you, that I won't survive the trial. He reminded me the trial wasn't mine to survive. I told him you torment me, he kept probing me, asking me what it was you tormented me about. But all I told him was I wished I'd gone to the police sooner, then things would have been different.

Today we're having an end-of-week play rehearsal in the Great Hall. I've read *Lord of the Flies* over a dozen times now. It's comforting. Reading about other children in circumstances that scare them, acting in ways they thought they never could, or would.

I carry my rucksack carefully, a candle in a glass jar inside. Saskia has a cupboard full, I asked if I could have one for my room. I took two, one for MK as well as a thank you. I'm due to see her at lunch today, I'll give it to her then.

When most of us have arrived in the hall Miss Mehmet claps three times, waits for the chitter-chatter of thirty or so girls in the same room to cease.

'I hope you've all been busy learning your lines, we'll pick up where we left off last time, which was, let's see – oh yes, Piggy's death.'

'Aww.'

'Very good, Lucy, but let's save the dramatics for onstage, shall we?'

'Miss?'

'Yes, Phoebe?'

'Are we allowed our scripts?'

She sighs, rests both hands on her hips, her large breasts wobbling for a second or two before settling.

'No, you should all be well on your way to knowing your lines by now, and if you aren't, we've got Milly on hand to prompt.'

No. A word Phoebe hates to hear. That, and Milly.

'Hurry up, you lot, over there, on to the stage and put your phones away. Silly girls.'

The noise lifts as chairs are pushed back, the last handful of girls climbing up the steps to the stage. I approach Miss Mehmet, ask her where I should sit. She explains that for the actual performances I'll be onstage tucked behind the curtains, but that it's not necessary right now.

'Take a seat in the front row and follow the script, line by line, okay?'

When I look up at the stage I can tell from Phoebe's face she's dreading it, hasn't learnt her lines. She's sat on a chair, on the left-hand side of the stage, frantically scanning each page. Too late. Show time.

'Shh, everyone, we're about to begin. And action.'

This is Phoebe's cue, the opening of the scene. Her feet are crossed, pulled back under her chair, not still though, the right one dances, a continual nervous jig. The script now on the floor next to her. Tempting. I see her look down, then out to me. I hold her gaze for a second, enjoy her needing me, then say the first line.

'Without Piggy's glasses, Ralph is –'

'Unable to light the fire.'

She interrupts, finishes the sentence, continues on.

'Ralph calls a meeting by blowing the conch.'

'Saafi – you're Ralph, pretend to blow the conch.'

The girls who do know their lines, the majority, take over. Progress is good until it's Phoebe's turn again. She stumbles and mumbles, looks like a fool. Feels worse, I imagine.

'No, no, no,' comes the cry from Miss Mehmet. 'Phoebe, this is unacceptable, what makes you so busy and important you can't learn your lines? I've watched Milly, she's hardly even using the script, knows the whole thing by heart.'

Ouch.

'I do know my lines, Miss, I just keep forgetting them.'

'Well it's not good enough. If you continue like this I'll be forced to give your part to Milly, understood?'

She nods, is silent, wouldn't dare say what she thinks to a teacher's face. When we finish, are filing out of the hall, she comes up behind me, whispers in my ear.

'And then Piggy dies.'

I have lunch with MK in her room today and I notice we both chose the same sandwich, ham and cheese. When we finish, she stands up, clips paper on to one of the easels and says, 'Feel free to start sketching whenever you like.'

I take the candle out of my bag.

'This is for you.'

'Me? Why?'

'To say thanks for helping me with the girls.'

'That's very sweet, Milly, but we're not allowed to accept presents from pupils unless it's Christmas.'

'It'll be half-term soon, Christmas isn't too long after that.'

I smile at her, walk over to her desk, put the candle down.

'It's vanilla. I tried to find a lavender one, I know you'd have liked that.'

She picks it up, smells it, then puts it back on the desk.

'It's lovely, but really I can't –'

'It's fine, it was a silly thing to do. Bin it if you like.'

I walk over to the easel, sit down.

'Don't be upset, Milly, it was a lovely thought, but rules are there for a reason.'

The phone on her desk rings, the noise, shrill, at odds with the sombre atmosphere in the room, a welcome intruder. She picks it up.

'Hello.'

A pause then, 'Yes, she's with me. Right now? Okay, I'll send her down,' and she replaces the receiver.

'Mrs Newmont's in reception.'

'What? Why?'

'Not sure, that was Mrs McDowell from the office, you should go and find out though.'

Bad news. Bad enough for Saskia to come to school.

'About the candle, Milly –'

'It's fine, I understand.'

I wouldn't want a present from me either.

Saskia smiles as I approach her in reception. She wouldn't smile, would she, if it was something really bad? Something about me?

'There you are.'

'Why are you here?'

'Mike called, asked me to pick you up, he's on his way home. June's back from holiday, I think she needs to talk to you about something. Have you got everything?'

I nod.

'I've signed you out, let's go.'

I follow tight leggings, bony hips, to the car. While I was making her a pot of tea the other night Mike came in for his eye drops. I watched him tilt his head. Squeeze. Drop. Blink. The sequence reminded me of you. You loved to teach me about chemistry, reactions that hurt. The hours you spent trawling the internet, learning. Eye drops for eyes become poison in tea. Taught me too. You didn't only want a helper, you wanted someone to carry on your work.

When we arrive home Saskia says, 'I should think they're already in the study, would you like me to come with you?'

'No, it's fine, it's probably better if it's just me and Mike.'

'I understand, I'll be around if you need me.'

I ignore Rosie jumping at my legs, eager and gooey for company during the day. My shoes echo on the marble, lonely as I walk, my heart pounds. Why is June here? The door to the study is open, I go in. Mike stands, a mistake, too formal, his face tense. Runs his hands through his hair.

'Hi, Milly,' says June.

'What's going on?' I ask.

'Take a seat, we'll talk everything through.'

'I don't want to sit down.'

Mike comes over to me.

'Sit next to me on the sofa.'

I don't have a choice, June's in my chair, the velvet cushion next to her. Mine.

'Shall I, Mike? Or do you want to?'

'You start.'

'Okay. I received a phone call this morning from Simon Watts, one of the lawyers.'

Skinny.

'There's a couple of things I need to tell you and I wanted to do it face-to-face and as soon as possible in case the papers get wind of anything. The first thing is that you'll definitely be cross-examined during the trial. As we expected, the defence want to focus on the most recent events, so the last few days you spent at home with your mother, including Daniel's death. They want to clarify a few things.'

'Clarify what?' I ask.

'I'm afraid we don't know. Simon did say it's likely to be a bit of smoke and mirrors, that the defence are playing the hype game. Sadly, we see these tactics all too often in the run-up to a trial.'

My left eyelid begins to tic, a hidden puppet master pulling on my strings. Reminding me you're still in charge.

'Surely we'll find out before the trial though, June?' Mike asks.

'Unless new evidence needs to be submitted, no, it's unlikely we'll find out exactly what it is the defence are referring to until we get to it. It could be as simple as Milly clarifying something she saw or heard. Our lawyers are confident nothing new will be brought up at trial.'

But they don't know you, do they? They don't know how your mind works. How much you enjoy playing with people.

'So what exactly will Milly be required to do?'

'She'll have to present twice. Once for the prosecution to question her and a second time for the defence. It's important to remember, Milly, that special measures can be reinstated at any point, it's not necessary for you to be questioned in the courtroom.'

'That may not be a bad idea, considering we're not sure what the defence are going to ask. What do you think, Milly?' Mike turns his body fully towards me.

'I don't know. I still want to do it, I need to, but I'm scared.'

'What are you scared of?'

'That she wants people to blame me.'

'Nobody's going to blame you, Milly.'

'You don't know that, you're not the jury.'

'No, we're not the jury,' June responds. 'But the court will recognize you as a minor, at home with her under duress, and to make things easier our lawyers have put together some example questions for you and Mike to go through.'

She makes it sound so simple. Like learning my ABC. But there's nothing simple about what I'm going to have to do in court.

'And will she have a chance to go through her statement again?'

'Yes, absolutely. In the week prior to the trial I'll ask you to bring Milly into court so she can have a look round and also review her statement. Once is more than enough – it can be very traumatizing to have to go over it all again and can also create doubt and confusion in witnesses. Can make them feel under pressure to "learn" their statement, when really we encourage them to focus on the questions they'll be asked.'

Mike responds by saying, 'That makes sense I suppose. We can go through this all again later, Milly, but is there anything you'd like to ask at this point?'

'No.'

Like Phoebe with Miss Mehmet, nothing I can say out loud.

'Will I be able to go into the courtroom with her, June?'

'I doubt it, no, in a high-profile case such as this one the judge will likely use what's called an anonymity order with the fewest number of people there possible. In the past there have been incidents of information from the court-room being leaked to the press. I'll be there the whole time, sat to the side of Milly. Yourself, and Saskia, if she wants, can wait in one of the family rooms nearby.'

'You said there were a couple of things you wanted to tell me, what was the other thing?'

'The date of the trial has been moved. The case that was due to be heard before ours has collapsed, which frees up the judge,' June explains. 'It's been brought forward, which means it'll start three weeks on Monday.'

Forty-five becomes twenty-four. I'm good at maths, especially when it involves you.

'The week after half-term,' I hear myself say. 'I won't be ready.'

'We'll make sure you are. June, is there anything else we can be doing in the meantime so Milly does feel ready?'

'Strange as this might sound, nothing hugely different from what you're doing now. Keep meeting on a weekly basis, more if either of you feel it's needed, and once I get back to the office I'll forward on to you the lawyers' questions.'

'So other than going through the questions, we continue as is?'

'That's right. Actually, will you be around over half-term? That'll probably be when Milly reviews her statement.'

'Yes, we will be. Phoebe's away with the school and we might head off for a few days, a bit of distraction, nowhere too far though so we can be around whenever you need us to be.'

'Good idea to take some time out, lie low for a bit. The news that the trial has been pushed forward will be released to the press tomorrow and, as we've previously discussed, we need to think about managing your exposure to this, Milly. Are any of the girls at school mentioning the case at all?'

I could tell the truth, that Mike's darling daughter likes to read you out loud, thinks you should be burned at the stake, an adoring audience nodding in agreement at her feet. But I don't want him to know how bad things are between me and Phoebe. I know who'll be shown the door.

So I say no, nobody really is.

'Grand. It's difficult I know but the right way to deal with it if they do is just to move yourself away. I'm aware this is an awful lot to take in but you're in excellent hands with Mike and if you think of anything you'd like to ask me after I leave, get Mike to pick up the phone or drop me an email. Okay?'

She approaches me, is about to touch my shoulder, withdraws her hand at the last minute when she remembers. She kneels down in front of me, the smell of stale coffee on her breath. 'It won't be as bad as you think it might be,' she says.

I look down at her. Committed, she is. Clueless though. *It won't be as bad as you think it might be — no, June, it'll be worse.*

After Mike sees her out, I tell him I want to be alone, I need time to process everything.

'Of course, yes, I'm here whenever you're ready to touch base.'

I stand at the sink in my bathroom. The razor on my skin. Press harder than usual. A knife through butter. A lightning bolt along my rib. Warm, red drips.

But no comfort.

I barely slept. Every time I closed my eyes I could see you, in your cell. You were smiling, happy with how things are going. How your plan is coming together. I start a count-down, in charcoal, inside the bathroom cabinet mounted on the wall. The days until the trial. I thought it would help, but when I write the number my hands begin to shake. Lawyers and jury members. The judge.

And you. There behind a screen.

Waiting.

Mike texted me first thing this morning saying he was going to work early, a full day of clients, but he'd like to catch up tomorrow, or Monday. There's nothing he can say or do. He's said it already, 'the only way out is through'.

Phoebe turns her back towards me as I enter the kitchen, butters two slices of toast. Saskia by the sink. A spare part.

'Morning,' she says.

'Hi, I just wanted to let you know I'm going out this afternoon, taking photos for art.'

'Fine,' she replies. 'I'll be out and about too, but perhaps we can all watch a movie together later on? Something girly.'

'I'm going straight to Clondine's after breakfast so you can count me out – not that you care,' Phoebe responds, throwing her knife in the sink and walking out, toast in her hand.

'What about you, Milly? Do you fancy it?'

'Maybe, but I'm not sure how long I'll be out for.'

I eat my breakfast alone, thankful I'm seeing Morgan later. In her messages she tells me how she dreams about living somewhere else, away from the estate. I've written a message to her a hundred times, deleted it before sending. I think if I ever told her about you it would be face-to-face.

We meet in the afternoon as arranged, down one of the side streets, away from the main road. She nods as I approach, a swift upwards movement of her head, a huge grin on her face.

'All right,' she says. 'Have you missed me?'

I smile which she takes as my reply.

'Come on,' she says, 'let's go.'

'Where are we going?'

'To meet some friends of mine.'

'Which friends?'

'Just a couple of boys I know.'

'Do we have to?'

'What's the problem?'

'Nothing, it doesn't matter.'

We cut through two streets I've never been along before. Quiet, the mayhem of the weekend markets not noticeable from here. The houses become less white, less grand, and soon we're near another estate. As we turn the corner and go to cross the road I see the line of black cars before I notice the church. A small group of people file out of the building, a vicar at the front, head bent down. A woman being supported, two men, one on either side.

'Wait, let them get in the cars, Morgan.'

'Nah, it's fine, come on.'

As we get closer I see the coffin, the brown varnished wood shining through the hearse window, the October sun penetrating the glass. A floral tribute. DAD. The drivers of the cars open the doors, smart in their uniforms, hats held by their side. I stop before we reach them. Interrupting their procession, their grief, feels wrong. Morgan walks on, oblivious, weaves her way through the mourners. When the cars are full and pull away, and the vicar goes back inside, I stand outside the church for a minute or two longer, think about my dad. He left long before the worst of it but he must have seen the news, he must know. Run away. Hide. Denial about who he married, denial about who you preferred over him.

Morgan whistles and beckons to me, looks impatient. When I join her she asks me why I stopped.

'Out of respect, I suppose.'

She spits on the ground, pulls a face that implies she doesn't get it or doesn't give a shit. A small pocket of heat flares up inside me. Lessons, she needs to be taught, I'm a good teacher.

We turn a corner into a residential street, tower blocks on both sides, a shop on the right, metal grating covering the windows. We enter the estate on our left, walk through it until we reach a small play park, the ground littered with glass and fast-food wrappers. No children playing, just two older boys sitting on the roundabout, cans of beer in their hands.

'All right, dickheads,' Morgan says.

'Shut up, you little shit,' replies one of the boys, a cap on his head, a gold stud in his right ear.

Morgan jumps on the roundabout, takes the can from his hand, gulps, burps afterwards, which makes them laugh. The other boy, inflamed spots on his neck, yellow heads on some of them, says, 'Who's this?'

'That's Milly, she's from opposite my bit.'

'Not bad,' he says. 'Come and sit next to me, make friends.'

'I'm all right,' I reply, taking a seat on the bench to the side of them.

'Too good for us, are you?'

I smile, try not to look fazed.

'You going to give me a beer or what?' Morgan asks.

'What do I get in return?' the boy with the cap replies.

'The pleasure of my dazzling company, of course.' Morgan stands up, takes a theatrical bow.

Cap boy is called Dean, his friend calls him that as he says, 'I bet I know what you'd really like.'

'Tell me about it,' he replies.

They light cigarettes, offer me one.

'No thank you.'

'Proper uptight, aren't you?'

Dean pulls Morgan towards him, starts to tickle her. She resists at first, then after he whispers something into her ear, she says, bet you I would, and walks off with him. Disappears into a small wooden play hut, painted in primary colours, names and graffiti scratched into the top. I try to steady the dread building in my stomach. Dirty and bad, the things happening to her. I want to go over to the hut, help her, but sometimes trying to help, doing something good, can end up meaning you do something bad.

Dean's friend moves to sit next to me, his fingernails ragged. Chewed. He positions his arm behind me, running along the back of the bench, touches my shoulder with his hand.

Touches me.

I try to ignore the movement I hear from the hut, bodies shifting into position. Morgan, my friend, on her knees or her back. The boy's face leans into my neck, the sounds from the hut replaced with the sound of his saliva as he moves a piece of gum around his mouth. I shiver, should stand up, can't feel my legs. Stuck.

'Are you cold? I'll warm you up.'

The smell of alcohol, the cigarette in his hand, the closeness of his face to mine takes me there.

To you.

A shadow, a canopy woven out of twisted love and lust, suffocated me in my bed every night. You.

He stubs out his cigarette on the wood of the bench between us. Flicks it on to the ground, a graveyard of butts. Bent into strange positions, necks broken, bodies folded.

He rests his hand on my thigh, moves it a little, further and further up. The word 'no' lodges in my throat, won't launch. Can't say it, doesn't work anyway. No meant yes, meant you always got what you wanted. Took it anyway. When his lips touch my neck they don't feel like they belong to him, they feel like someone else's. I never wanted to be touched like that. I never wanted you to touch me like that.

'Get off, get the fuck off me,' I say, and jump up.

'Jesus, what's your fucking problem?'

I walk over to the hut, hammer on the roof, each step I take punctuated with images of being back in our house, in your room.

'Morgan. Morgan. Let's go, I want to go now.'

The boy in the hut calls me a freak. A cock block. A bitch. The sound of a zip going up.

'Chill out, I'll be there in a minute,' Morgan replies.

I hurry up the slope away from them, towards the parked cars, a black cat underneath. Eyes closed, peaceful. Lucky if it walks in front of me. It doesn't. I'm angry, angry with Morgan. Nobody made her, she went into the hut smiling, still is as she walks towards me now. A can of beer in one hand, takes a mouthful, gargles, then spits it out. Dirty.

'Why were you freaking out?'

'I want to go home.'

'Fucking hell, as if you've never done anything like that.'

I don't reply, I don't know how to explain.

'Can I come home with you? You could sneak me in on the balcony.'

Yes, is what I should say. She needs looking after, out of harm's way. She needs to behave better. I could help her do that.

'So, can I?'

'Yes.'

You coach me as we walk back to the house, ideas on how to teach Morgan, how to 'help' her be clean, but what you're saying frightens me, it doesn't feel good to hear. I don't want to do that to her, she's all I've got, she's my only friend. I need her. And that's why I do it, when she kneels down by a row of parked cars to tie her shoelace, I look. Usually I wouldn't, usually I don't want to be reminded, but this time I stare in the car window. Your face, the spit of mine, stares back. ACCEPT WHO YOU ARE, ANNIE. 'I don't want to,' I reply.

'Who are you talking to?' Morgan asks as she stands up.

I shake my head, she smiles and calls me nuts, says, don't worry about what happened in the park, they're dickheads anyway. And I realize, you can say what you want to the lawyers about me, you already have, I'm sure, but Morgan is mine. I get to decide. I tell her I've changed my mind, too risky to sneak her in with Saskia around. She's annoyed, says she'll have to go home now and be hassled by her little brother and sister. Thanks a lot, Mil, she says, before she walks off.

I want to tell her, she's welcome. But she wouldn't understand.

17

The questions are straightforward when Mike asks me them. He's a psychologist, programmed to support and hold me up, not like defence lawyers though.

He reads them out. What exactly did you see through the peephole on the night Daniel Carrington died? How long did you stand at the peephole for? Are you sure that's what you saw your mother doing? You're absolutely sure? What happened after that?

Please tell the court again. And again.

When we finish he tells me I did really well. He places the page of questions down and says he's sorry I'm having to go through this. That it must feel very exposing, the idea of answering questions in front of a jury and a judge. Yes, it is, I tell him, it's scary not knowing what might happen on the day. What might be said. But I'll be okay, I think that going to court, facing you, is my way of helping the children you hurt. My way of taking responsibility. He talks about survivor's guilt and how it can make a person feel more culpable than they are. Sometimes I think you feel like that, that the deaths of the children were your fault. Am I right, he asks? I'm not sure, I reply, sometimes, yes. You did nothing wrong, he says, and if your mother says anything to the contrary, it's her attempt to continue abusing you.

A neat explanation, a ribbon in a bow.

We talk about the time you drove us to Manchester

during the school holidays. You were careful, so careful, to spread what you did over great distances. The underground network of desperate women who were sufficiently re-assured by you to hand over a child. Groomed from afar for years. The camouflage again was me, a daughter of your own. We could have gone on and on like that but then you took Daniel, someone I knew. Too close to home.

'What would you say now to your younger self that would have comforted you then?'

'I don't know.'

'You have to try. What would you have liked to hear?'

That I was different from you.

'That one day it would stop.'

'You made it stop, you were very brave to go to the police.'

'I waited too long, too many bad things had happened already.'

'If you could've been heard earlier, what would you have said?'

'Help me. Leave me alone.'

'How could you have been helped if you wanted to be left alone?'

'I don't know, it's just how I feel.'

'Frightened, I think. What about if you'd said, "Help me, take me somewhere safe"?'

I count the books on the shelves. Numbers help. Then I begin to cry, hide my face with the cushion. Mike sits quietly, lets me cry, then says, 'You do deserve that, Milly, you deserve to be safe and to have a new life.'

I remove the cushion. His face is so open, looks at me. He wants to make it better for me, I can tell, but he doesn't get it.

'You don't get it, Mike. You think you know me but you don't.'

'I think I'm getting to know you, I think I know you better than most people. Wouldn't you agree?'

If that was true, he'd know what to say. He'd know that the best way to help me is to say I can stay. That he'll look after me. But I'm too scared to ask him. I know once the trial's finished I'll have to leave. Start over. And there's nothing I can do about it.

'Can we stop, Mike? It's been over an hour. I'm tired, I want to go to bed.'

He senses shutdown, knows to take his foot off the gas for tonight.

'Okay, let me grab your night-time meds.'

I stash the pills with the others, open up my laptop to see if there's anything about you in the news. You've been placed into solitary confinement, no details other than an attempted attack by a fellow prisoner following the announcement your trial has been moved forward. Protecting you matters, I imagine, the public pressure to keep you alive.

Make you pay.

18

Dirt on my hands, a towel in the sink. Mike should have left me where he found me late last night after our session. The dark of the cellar.

Phoebe's on the landing when I come out of my room, balanced on the edge of the banister, head in her phone, one foot on the carpet. Perfectly painted toenails, in pink. She looks up as I pass, says, what was all the noise about last night, you woke me up. I reply with the first thing that comes into my head.

'I had a stomach ache, Mike brought me some tablets.'

'Yeah, well, next time, keep it down.'

I continue past her, down one flight of stairs, turn and ask.

'How are your lines for the play coming along?'

She gives me the finger, mouths fuck you. She knows Mike and Saskia are around, could easily hear.

'Let me know if I can help,' I reply, smiling.

She pushes off the banister, storms into her room, kicking the door shut behind her.

Saskia's at the kitchen table nursing a large mug, fingers thin, clasped round it, pronounced veins running up her knuckles to her wrists. She greets me with good morning, a faraway look in her eyes, more of a pleasantry than a genuine attempt at conversation.

'Eggs?' Mike offers, a wooden spoon in one hand.

He wears an apron with James Bond on the front, 'licence

to grill' written underneath. He sees me looking, laughs a little, tries to mask his concern. The inadequacy he must be feeling. Even after our session, I'm still fucked up.

'Saskia bought it for my birthday last summer, didn't you, Sas?'

'What's that?'

'The apron.'

'Yes, darling, I think so.'

I look at Mike as he turns back to the stove top. Tall. His body, strong and fit, his hair sandy, streaked with grey. The weight of us all on his broad shoulders, though I've never heard him complain once.

'Here you go,' he says. 'Scrambled eggs.'

I thank him and sit down next to Saskia.

'Aren't you having any?' I ask.

'No, no, I like to eat later.'

Or not at all. Mike goes into the hallway, stands on the first step, shouts to Phoebe. He has to shout twice for her to come out of her room and reply.

'I'll be down in a minute.'

He joins us at the table, dig in, he says, go on. He asks me if I have any idea what I'd like to do for half-term.

'I don't mind, I'm happy to stay here. I know you're both busy.'

'I think June was right the other day, we should take some time out. There's a nice spot in the country we've been to before, the trees will be beautiful this time of year.'

'Well, this is cosy, isn't it?' Phoebe says as she walks in.

'Morning, grab some eggs, join us.'

'What was going on last night? You woke me up.'

'I already told Phoebe about the stomach ache I had, how you brought me some pills.'

Mike hesitates, it's not in his nature to lie but he'll rationalize it in his head. Protective. A necessity.

'I didn't hear a thing,' Saskia says.

Nobody looks surprised.

'Yeah, well, it took me ages to get back to sleep.'

'Sorry, Phoebs,' soothes Mike. 'Anyway, we were just discussing half-term, it's a shame you can't come with us.'

'Tramping about in a wood in the middle of nowhere, no thanks. I'd much rather go to Cornwall with my friends, thank you very much.'

Devon's near Cornwall. It used to be home.

'Lots of woods there too, you know,' Saskia says.

It's not a bad attempt, verging on funny, but Phoebe doesn't think so, turns her back, fills a glass with water from the tap. I see Mike's hand move off the table, rest on Saskia's thigh. A captain of a shaky ship, he is. Mutiny possible. Likely.

'You need to eat something, Phoebs.'

'Nah, not hungry, I'm on a diet.'

'Not first thing in the morning you aren't, you need breakfast.'

'Why? I don't see Mummy dearest having any.'

'She's not spending the whole day at school or captaining a hockey team, is she?'

Phoebe mumbles into the lip of the glass, no, she's not doing anything as per usual.

'At least grab a cereal bar from the cupboard then, eat it at break.'

'Fine,' she says. 'Whatever.'

Phoebe and me leave together, no choice, Mike and Saskia wave us off. We split company the next house down. I watch her long lean body as she crosses the road, walks with confidence, a world away from what's on the inside. A couple of weeks ago I went down to the laundry to get a clean towel, heard voices. Sevita doing the ironing, Phoebe cross-legged on the floor doing homework. Sevita looked up as I walked in, smiled, hello, Miss Milly. Phoebe's face said it all, angry. Jealous. Didn't want me to be there, didn't want to share. What she can't get from Saskia, she finds elsewhere, needs it.

Passing the tower blocks reminds me that I forgot to tell Mike and Saskia I'll be late home from school. I send them both a text letting them know I'm helping with props for the play, should be back by six or seven. A lie, a little one, the colour white. I'm looking forward to seeing Morgan again. I looked after her at the weekend, I sent her home. I haven't been able to shake the idea of telling her about you, not all of it, but enough so I'd be able to talk about it if I wanted to. June wouldn't approve. I was given a new identity so I would feel protected. Invisible. Nobody would know who I am. London's a huge city, she said, you'll be just another face in the crowd. What's most important, she said, is you never tell anybody who you are, or anything about your mum. Do you understand how important that is? Yes was my answer, still is, but I never realized how lonely it would be.

The day drags. German, then music. Maths and art. MK's not my teacher. I think about her spending time with other girls, talking. Laughing with them. I sent her another email yesterday asking if I could come and see her but she hasn't replied.

Biology, the last lesson of the day. Dissection. The heart of a pig. Human the same, almost. Ventricles. The atrium, the mighty vena cava. I know a lot about a person's insides.

Glorious in their redness, fifteen hearts laid out on the bench as we arrive, one for each girl. Prof West, a little bit blind, a little bit old, tells us to follow the instructions on the white board at the front of the class.

Knives at the ready.

Slice we do, a cut here, a snip there. A struggle for some, easier for me. I'm the first one finished. I stare at the heart, now in pieces, spread out in a silver tray. Two bloody scalpels and a pair of tweezers to blame. I listen to the comments around me. Gross. Eww, I hate biology, can't wait to give it up next year. Help me with mine. No way, I can hardly do my own. Bleugh.

I put my hand up. It takes a minute or two for Prof West's bald head to look up, survey the class.

'I'm finished, sir.'

'Wash your hands then, and write up your observations.'

After I've finished at the sink I walk back to my bench, turn to a new page in my exercise book, start to write, but then I hear them. Clondine and Izzy giggling, the row in front of me looking over their shoulders at me. They turn away when I look. I start writing again. Then it happens.

A heart on my face.

Bounces off my left cheek, lands on my breast, drops to the floor. My lab coat already removed. I touch my hand to my face. Sticky. Blood on my fingers. Izzy films me, Clondine keeps watch though Prof's no threat. I turn away from them. My shirt's stained, a bleed from the heart belongs to the pig, could easily be mine.

'Time to tidy up,' says Prof West.

'I'm not finished, sir,' comes a voice from the front.

'Time waits for no man or woman, Elsie, you should have worked faster.'

I'd move if I could, yet I can't feel my legs. Can't. Feel. I'll always be a freak to them. I know Prof's coming this way, I can hear his shoes. Brown leather brogues, polishes them daily I bet. He stops in front of me.

'For heaven's sake, child, what have you been up to? You said you were finished and now you've got blood all over your shirt and your face. Get cleaned up and for goodness' sake pick that heart up off the floor.'

I hear the snorts of stifled laughter as Prof West continues on past.

Zoe, a girl on the same bench as me, a witness but silent, bends down, uses a paper towel to pick up the heart, hands me another for my face. Took the time to wet it for me. She points to where I need to wipe.

I nod, thank her, wishing I was young enough for someone to do it for me. Clondine and Izzy flash sarcastic smiles at me as we file out of the lab. The corridors are busy but space is made for me as I approach. Is that blood on her shirt? I think so, yuck. I use the science-block toilets to change into the jeans and hoodie I hid in my bag earlier this morning. No uniforms on the estate, especially not one from this school. My phone rings. I kneel down and retrieve it from my rucksack. It's Morgan checking I'm still coming, and when I notice a familiar make-up bag abandoned on the floor of the next-door cubicle, I tell her I'll be there in about twenty minutes, there's something I have to do first.

When I arrive on the tower block roof she's smoking a cigarette, says, 'There's a bird over there, I think its wing's all fucked up.'

'Where?'

'Over there.'

She points to a crate, and says, 'I covered it up with that, it was flapping about all over the place, freaking me out.'

I walk over, crouch down, look through the gaps in the plastic. Honeycomb-shaped gaps. A pigeon, one wing hanging low. Broken. Its head moves fast, a continual bobbing. I don't know why I do it, but I rattle the crate, a flurry of panic from inside, it begins to coo. An SOS to its friends, fly away, Peter, fly away, Paul. It would join them if it could, but it can't, it's been caught. Morgan squats next to me, asks me what I'm doing. I lift the crate up at one side, reach my hand in and grab the bird. Hard. I hold it into the ground, a tiny thud reverberates against my fingers. Broken wing, not heart. Not yet. It begins to coo again, calls to the others. Beady eyes and bobbing heads hidden on rooftops, the baby birds watch too, the adults make them.

I do it quickly, it's the kind thing to do.

'Fuck, that's gross, why did you do that? Jesus.'

She looks away.

'It would have been worse if I hadn't. It would have died slowly all on its own.'

'We could have taken it to a vet or something.'

'It was in pain, but it's not any more. I helped it.'

'Rather you than me.'

Yes.

I place the crate over it again and we go back to the vent, lie down like statues on the cold ground, the sky awash with noise from aircraft as they roar overhead to Heathrow. Beam me up, Scotty, anywhere will do. Morgan lights another cigarette, blue fingers of smoke move in swirls, stroking the air above us. Witches' breath.

'Why so quiet, not got any stories for me today?'

Only one, but I'm not sure I should tell it.

'Not really, no.'

'Great company you are. I can't stay for very long, my uncle's here, he's dead strict.'

Just a few more minutes please, let me get it right in my head before I say it out loud. My mother is. No. Have you seen the news, the woman that. No. Fuck. What am I doing? I'm not supposed to tell anyone.

'What's up with you today?' she asks.

'Nothing, why?'

'You've made your finger bleed. Look.'

'Sorry.'

'No need to be sorry, but if you've got something to say, just spit it out.'

It's like skating on a frozen lake. It looks safe, feels safe, but somebody has to go first, test it out to see if the ice will hold. She likes me, we're friends. I can tell her, not all of it, some of it though. Can't I?

'If you're not going to talk, I'm off. I'd rather watch telly than sit in silence.'

'Wait.'

'Fuck's sake, what's your problem?'

It's getting dark on the roof, just me and her. Nobody else is here, nobody else has to know. She likes me. I'm nothing like you. She'll understand. Won't she?

'If I told you something would you still want to be my friend?'

'Yeah, I reckon we can tell each other anything, can't we?'

I nod because it's true, she texts me most nights, asks if I'm getting any hassle from Phoebe and not to worry, she's got my back.

'What is it you want to tell me?'

'I'm not sure I should.'

'You can't start then not finish.'

'I shouldn't have said anything in the first place.'

'Well you have now and I'm not leaving until you do.'

Rules are made to be . . . Aren't they?

'Mil, you're starting to piss me off, I have to go soon.'

'Just promise you'll still be my friend.'

'Okay, whatever, I promise. Now tell me.'

I sit up, use my foot to hook a strap of my rucksack, pull it towards me. She sits up too. I ask for her lighter, too dark to see it without. I remove the newspaper clipping, the one I rescued from the common room, from the front pocket of my bag, smooth it out on my jeans. Risky carrying it every day I know, all it would take would be for Phoebe or Izzy to empty my bag, their manicured nails unfolding the seams across your face. My face and yours, so alike.

'What is it?' she asks.

I contemplate backing out, burning it instead of showing it to her, but I'm not sure I could hold a flame to your face. The first time I flick the lighter, it blows out.

'I didn't see, do it again.'

The second time, it lights up your face, your mouth and your lips. You can't see it in the photo, but there's a freckle that sits to the right of your chin.

This time she sees who it is.

'What the fuck! That's that woman who's been in the news, the one that killed the kids.'

'Yeah.'

'Why are you showing her to me?'

The lighter goes out. Why am I? Push. Pull. The damaged things damaged people do. I was sure when I left the toilets at school that telling Morgan was an okay thing to do. That she'd feel differently about me, not like the girls in my year. I know what they'd say, how they'd feel. But they're not my friends, she is, and I long to hear her say the words: you are nothing like your mother.

I ask her what she thinks about it, about you.

'What do you mean, what's to think? She's a psycho, clearly. Why do you care?'

'What if it was someone you knew?'

'As if. Don't get me wrong, there's a lot of shit goes on in the estate, but nothing like that.'

She promised she'd still be my friend, I can tell her.

'What if it was someone I knew?'

'Nice try, it's October though, not April Fool's.'

A greedy feeling of relief lapping at my heels, tempting me. Of being able to release some of the burden of you.

'Watch,' I tell her.

I hold the clipping next to my face and light the flame again.

'Watch what?'

'Just look at her face, then look at mine.'

She moves in for a closer look.

'Shit,' she replies. 'You look really like her, eww.'

'That's what I've been trying to tell you.'

'What?'

'I look like her because. Because.'

Please don't leave when I tell you.

'What? Because she's your long-lost aunt or something?'

'No, it's not my aunt, it's my mum.'

I let the flame go out, fold up the picture, put you back in my bag. I can feel Morgan staring at me, waiting for the punchline, but there isn't one. She's the first to speak.

'Tell me you're joking.'

She knows by my lack of reply, I'm not.

'Holy fuck,' she says.

I can't help it, tears begin to brim in my eyes. She gets up, takes a step away from me.

'Don't go yet, please.'

'I have to, my uncle will be mad.'

She's lying, she's leaving because she's scared.

'You said you'd still be my friend, you promised.'

'It's not like that, it's just a lot to take in, you know.'

Yes, I do. It was a lot for me too.

'Is that why you're in a foster family?'

I nod.

'Do they know about her?'

'Mike and Saskia do, not Phoebe, and the headmistress at school, she knows.'

'Nobody else?'

'No.'

'Not being funny, but why did you tell me?'

'I've wanted to tell you for a while, it felt wrong keeping it secret from you.'

'For real it's your mum?'

'Yes.'

'Jesus, she needs to be put down, all those kids she took were about the same age as my little brother and sister.'

I nod again. What she says is true, you do need putting down, yet it hurts to think about it happening.

'Tell me you weren't living with her?'

'I wasn't, I lived with my dad until he died. I haven't seen her for years.'

The lie slips out easily, and she doesn't question it. If she reads that there was a child living at home with you I'll tell her I don't know who it was, that it must have been someone you'd taken in at some point.

'Thank fuck you haven't seen her for years. How did they catch her?'

'Not sure, somebody at work I think.'

Not true. Somebody much closer to home. The biggest betrayal of all when blood hands in blood. Families are supposed to stick together, birds of a feather, but I want to fly in a different flock, to a different place.

'She got what was coming, I guess.'

'I guess so, yeah.'

'I have to go,' she says.

'Okay.'

She walks towards the door, I call out to her.

'Morgan.'

'Yeah?'

She walks back over to me, I stand up and ask, 'Has it made you feel differently about me?'

'Not really, no. It's not your fault, Mil. Nobody should blame you for what your mum did. Anyway, you're nothing like her.'

'Do you mean that?'

'Yeah.'

Thank you.

19

Last week, sat in the alcove, Mike talking to June on the phone. Just before he hung up, he said, it's the calm before the storm. I knew what he meant, he was right, the past week has been very calm. Outwardly. After the initial reporting of the trial date being moved, there hasn't been much mention of you in the press. The journalists are resting, gearing up for the trial to begin, only ten days from now. You, also resting, saving your strength. You've only come to me twice. Both times you said nothing but laid your scaly body across my neck. I couldn't breathe or move, the weight of concrete. The weight of our secrets.

When I saw Morgan over the weekend I wasn't sure how she would be. Whether she'd have changed her mind, decided she didn't like me any more, but she was the same as before. She likes to talk about you though, about what you did, which is harder than I thought it would be because it's not just your story, it's mine.

June came over on Wednesday evening while Saskia took Phoebe and Izzy out for dinner. She and Mike went over the lawyers' questions again. She kept saying I was doing grand, and how hard it must be to have to keep going over what happened, that it'll be easier once the trial's over. Mike didn't say much. Usually he would, he'd agree, but not this time. He sat and watched me closely, nodding every now and then. I didn't like the way it made me feel. A small seed of panic. Inside. Vulnerable. We ended the session with a game of cards. Blackjack. It's my favourite, Mike said. I didn't have the heart to tell him that although your version was different, it was your favourite too.

Today we break up for half-term. We have a play rehearsal all morning, it's a big deal, Miss Mehmet's words, not ours, because Ms James the headmistress is due to watch. When breakfast is over Mike insists on driving us both to school as he's going that way.

'Humour me,' he says, winking at Phoebe.

'Fine, all right, Dad. I just need to text Iz, tell her not to wait for me.'

Saskia smiles, says it reminds her of the school runs years ago. Phoebe ignores her, walks out to the car, sits up front next to Mike. He asks about the play, how things are going.

'Good, yeah, the rehearsal should be loads of fun today,' she replies.

'I'm sure it will be, we can't wait to come and see it.'

When we get to school we sign in at registration and head to the Great Hall. As soon as Miss Mehmet arrives she begins to fuss, she wants it to be perfect. She bosses around the technical crew, two external guys brought in to man the lights and stage effects. It's the first time we've used them and everybody laughs as a whoosh of smoke fills the stage in preparation for the pig-hunting scene. A few of the girls are missing, the art history trip to Paris left this morning, so Miss Mehmet asks me to step in as the pig. I don't like the idea of being hunted, but I can't say no in front of everyone.

'And, Phoebe, I know you're narrator but we need more bodies on stage for this scene so can you fill in as one of the boys.'

'Gladly,' she replies, looking at me.

'There should be a spear for everyone stage left by the props cupboard. Once you have one, on to the stage please and, Milly, there should also be a papier-mâché pig's head, grab that please.'

I know this scene inside out. It's a play, not real, but when I put on the pig's head it starts to feel real. Though light to carry, the head is large and, once on, hard to see out of. The only way not to trip is to look down at my feet. My breath comes in short shallow bursts, creating an intense heat that rebounds off my face, and back again. Through the layers of glue and paper, I hear Miss Mehmet.

'Milly, you'll be entering stage right with Jack and his gang closely behind, and remember, everyone, this is a key scene where we start to see real savagery emerging from the boys. Think blood, gore, and use the hunting chant to demonstrate this. Once I call for lights and smoke, Milly, you're on.'

The girls find it easy to get into role. Somebody to the right bangs their spear on the ground, a repetitive hammering that makes the lower part of my stomach contract. A voice on my left whispers, run, little piggy, run. You never called me piggy, but you often made me run. SO MUCH FUN WE USED TO HAVE, ANNIE, DIDN'T WE?

'Go on, you're on,' somebody says behind me.

I missed my cue, listening to you.

As soon as I step on to the stage I bend my knees, drop low, as pig-like as possible. My breathing is heavy, weighed down by you. There with me. The noise of the spears unites. *Thud, thud. THUD.* I smell the dry ice from the smoke machine, it swirls around my feet as the stage lights up with flashes of red, punctuated with strobe lighting. The chant begins.

'Kill the pig, cut her throat, spill her blood.'

Different words from yours, same intent.

Somebody bangs on a drum, the spears move closer, Jack and his boys. I move around the stage, it's supposed to be a chase.

'Kill the pig, cut her throat, spill her blood.'

Thud, thud. THUD.

I tried to find new places to hide, but you knew where to look.

'There it is,' a voice cries.

A high-pitched bow-wow like the noise a child makes playing cowboys and Indians lifts in the air, it's their signal. Time to attack. Me. I move into centre stage, stumble by mistake on to the floor, not safe on the floor. Not supposed to be, the pig doesn't make it out alive, remember? The strobe lights intensify, another release from the smoke machine.

'Kill the pig. Cut her throat. Spill her blood.'

The feet surrounding me stamp in time with their spears. The first jab happens fast, from behind, I can guess who it was. I roll on to my back. Spear after spear begins to nudge and prod me. The drum slows to a steady hypnotic rhythm, the chant lower, more menacing.

'Cut her throat, spill her blood,' another bow-wow released from the person on my left. A loud single beat on the drum calls them to silence. The sound of the papier-mâché head sucking in and releasing from my face, the only noise, I'm breathing so hard. The feet around me start to move in a circular motion, disorientate me further. I hated the mask you made me wear, the same feelings now. Can't. Breathe.

'This time, no mercy,' says Jack, played by Marie.

Her spear goes down to the right of me, hits the floor hard. To the audience, through the smoke and the strobes, it'll look like I've been speared through the heart. I'm carried off stage by my legs and my arms but here in my new life, without you in charge, I'm placed on my feet and nothing bad happens. I wish I could cheer and join in with the laughter and jokes backstage, but instead I go to the toilet in the dressing room, peel off the pig's head, splash my face with cold water, count backwards from fifty. The numbers slowly cast their spell, the flashbacks recede, and after a while I feel safe enough to leave.

As I come down the stairs from the stage, into the hall, Ms James is waiting for me. She invites me to take a seat at the front, away from the girls, she'd like a word.

'How are you enjoying your first play at Wetherbridge?'

'Good, thank you, Ms James.'

'You gave a very convincing performance, Milly, but I was a bit concerned to find out it was you playing the pig.'

'I'm not, I was standing in for Aimee, she's on the Paris trip.'

'I see, and I can also see it might have been tricky to say no, but still, you do need to be aware of situations that could trigger something unpleasant for you, given – you know.'

I want to put the pig's head back on and cry. There isn't a minute goes by at school when I don't feel reminded.

Given – you know.

'There's a couple of other things I wanted to chat to you about, Milly. Mr Newmont emailed me to let me know you'll be going to court, the week after next I believe.'

I nod.

'Have you been managing to concentrate at school?'

'Mostly, yes.'

'You're clearly very bright, Milly, so it's not a huge concern if you need to take some time away, we can arrange for work to be sent home to you.'

'I'd rather be busy, if that's okay.'

'Of course. But if you change your mind, just ping my PA an email and ask her to book an appointment for you to see me.'

'Thank you.'

'The other thing I wanted to talk to you about is Miss Kemp. I understand you've been spending a bit of time with her. The difficulty, Milly, is that Miss Kemp doesn't know about . . .'

She nods rather than says it, waits for me to nod back, show her I've understood, then continues.

'So we need to be careful, if you like. I'm aware you tried to give her a gift, which really is very sweet but not something we encourage – in fact, it's against school rules. However, in your particular case I can perhaps see where the confusion has come from.'

That's why she hasn't answered my emails.

'Miss Kemp is a wonderful teacher, very committed, but that said, one must be clear where one draws the line.'

'I'm not sure I understand what you mean, Ms James.'

'What I mean is, if you'd find it easier we can look at assigning you a new guidance teacher.'

'Why?'

'I've asked Mr Newmont to talk this over with you during half-term, I'm sure he will. Okay?'

'Yes, Ms James.'

'There's no need to look worried, we're all on your side and I'm sure we can work something out. How does that sound?'

Patronizing.

'Fine, thank you.'

'Great, keep up the excellent work with the play, no doubt it'll be a glorious performance on the night.'

I stand when she does, as we're expected to.

I wake up crying, halfway through the night. I dreamt I was in court.

When the defence lawyer turned round to face me he shrank to the size of a boy, asked me why I let you hurt him. Tears in his eyes.

I'm sorry, I said.

We don't believe you, said the jury in reply.

20

After school yesterday Mike told me he'd booked us two nights at a hotel, a place called Tetbury. We're going on Monday. He mentioned he'd like to catch up with me, about Miss Kemp, but it could wait until the weekend.

Phoebe and I are about to leave for Matty's party, the same one Joe mentioned on the bus. Mike agreed to let Phoebe go on the condition she took me too, plus, he added, if you go together, I'll let you walk home on your own. You wouldn't want me turning up at his door now, would you? Before we leave he reminds us our curfew is midnight, no later, and no drinking, okay?

'Yes, Dad, okay.'

Phoebe calls Izzy as soon as we leave the house, says it's a bummer she can't come, how much longer does she think she'll be grounded for. Izzy's reply makes her laugh and before she hangs up she says, don't worry, beatch, I'll tell you all about it tomorrow. Poor Izzy, she must have been delighted when Prof West returned her make-up bag, but not so when she realized he'd seen the cigarettes inside. No room to wriggle out of that one, her name written in Tipp-Ex on the bottom of the bag, left slightly open on Prof West's desk when his room was empty, all the hearts tidied away.

We arrive at another large white house and Phoebe rings the doorbell. A boy answers, tall, six foot, maybe more. He smiles when he sees who it is and says, 'Party is on.'

He holds out his hand to me.

'Matty.'

I shake it and say, hi, I'm Milly. I feel sick as he pulls open the door for us to walk in, music spills from the living room and as we enter I notice a table on the left. Bottles of spirits, a large glass bowl, some kind of punch.

'It's hardly very Halloween in here, is it, Matty?'

'Fuck off, Phoebs, my folks only left a couple of hours ago, they made me and Thom promise not to have any parties while they're away. Anyway, you're gross enough for ten Halloweens, no décor required.'

He ends his sentence with a ghoulish 'bahahaha' laugh.

'Shut up and get me a drink. So Thom's back from uni then?'

'Yep, supposed to be in charge but fucked off to catch up with his mates as soon as Mum and Dad left.'

'Is he coming back?'

'I see somebody's still got a crush on my bro then.'

'Hardly, just being friendly, that's all. Anyway, I like someone else.'

'Who?'

'Just some guy I met over the summer, he doesn't live in London though.'

'AKA doesn't exist, you mean. Here, I've made you a voddy.'

She takes the plastic tumbler from him, sinks into a sofa beside two girls I've never seen before, starts chatting to them.

'Would you like a drink?' he asks.

I say yes please because everybody else is holding one. I won't drink it though, wits, about me. I take a seat in the corner after he gives it to me. More and more people arrive.

They all know somebody who knows somebody, the rich private school network spins a web, reaches far and wide. Phoebe's on and off her phone, numerous calls. She kicks one of the boys at her feet, trying to distract her by doing a break-dancing move, the worm. Stop it, she mouths, and when she hangs up, the worm boy asks her, 'When will we get them?'

'When he comes, all right, knob-head.'

She kicks him again, although this time he grabs her leg, wrestles her to the floor. He sits astride her, hands round her throat. Everybody laughs but it doesn't look funny or fun to me. Clondine arrives with two older boys. Phoebe goes over to them and one of the boys puts his arm round her waist, pulls her into his body, she pushes him away, laughing.

'You'll be begging for it later, trust me,' he says.

She's about to respond when her phone rings, the call is quick, finished in seconds. When she hangs up, she shouts.

'Right, peeps, time to hand your cash over.'

Notes are gathered, passed round the room until they reach her, nobody asks what for.

'You too, don't think I don't see you there.'

I look away, hold my drink up to my mouth, pretend to take a sip.

'Maybe I'll get you to help me, that way if we get caught we're both in the shit.'

'Yeah, you should,' says one of the girls on the sofa.

Insignificant. Face like a hyena, laugh the same.

Phoebe looks at me and says, come on then, what you waiting for, don't say I never include you in anything. When we get to the front door she pauses before she opens it, looks at me and says, 'Tell Dad about this and I'll mess you up, got it?'

Got it.

At the door is a man in a black padded suit, a motorbike helmet in one hand. She doesn't kiss him but greets him by name, Tyson.

'Shit, hang on, someone's coming. Just say you're delivering pizzas if anyone asks. Oh, fuck's sake, it's fine, it's Joe.'

When he gets to the door, he says hi. Phoebe ignores him, he walks past us into the porch, smiles at me.

'Hey, Milly.'

He remembers my name.

'Hi.'

'How many do you want?' asks Tyson.

'Thirty, if you have them.'

'Thirty? Big night then.'

'Just broken up for half-term, you know how it goes.'

He nods, takes one of his leather gloves off, holds out his hand. Phoebe places the money in it, rolled like a cigar. He trusts her enough not to count, a regular thing maybe, walks down the driveway to his bike, parked at the kerb. He looks around before opening the top of the seat, takes a minute or two, and comes back holding a large brown paper bag.

'There's thirty inside,' he says as he approaches the door. 'And these are on me,' handing her a small bag of pills. 'New shit, guaranteed to make you fly.'

She smiles, blows him a kiss, you're the best, Tyson, totally the best. He looks pleased, I hear his bike before the door closes, a rev of the engine, long and sustained. We go back into the living room, the air hazy with smoke, ash being tapped into empty tumblers and bottles. Lazy drunk bodies, lying on chairs. Apathy revived by Phoebe's announcement.

'Party bags are here.'

I'm surprised to see she means it. She tips a load of children's party bags on to the table, a clown on the front of each one.

'Help yourselves, bitches.'

Like free bowls of sweets, nobody stays shy for long, the table of clowns demolished. A blink of an eye. Ever the drama queen, Phoebe clears her throat, waits for the full attention of the room, shakes the extra bag of pills Tyson gave her in the air. Rattles to babies, toothy, some adorned with brightly coloured metal braces. Whoop, double whoop, somebody says, time to get f-u-u-u-c-k-e-d up.

'What are they?' Clondine asks.

Phoebe takes a pill from the bag, moves it around between her fingers, examines it.

'It's got a Superman logo on it, Tyson said they'll make us fly.'

She pops one in her mouth, walks around the room delivering the rest into hands outstretched, as if she is god or queen of the teens. Bless me please.

A full circle done, a couple left in the bag still.

'Open wide, dog-face.'

'No,' I reply. 'No thank you,' I modify.

'Not sure I understand that word,' she says.

'Leave her be, Phoebe, all the more for us.'

Joe saunters by, an attempt at casual. I don't know boys, how they function, but his casual looks like concern, needs a bit more work. Phoebe turns away, bored of my face.

'Yeah, you're right, it would only be a waste, she's fucked up already.'

Her nails like talons, almond in shape, she flicks another pill down her throat. Lips pressed into a pout, close the moist cave. Dark. She misses the wink Joe gives me, a secret mutiny against her majesty. Off with his.

It doesn't take long. The perfectly smart and beautiful privileged crowd morph into a mob. Animals. Pack mentality. Outside in the garden, howl to the moon. Saucers for eyes, mouths a-judder. Smoking. One day these boys and girls will run the world, in the meantime, they ruin it.

I find a quiet space at the top of the stairs on the first landing, an abandoned party bag on the way. The contents, ingenious, the seductive way it's been put together, wrapped in foils, plastic tubes. I pretend it's Christmas, how it is in the movies, unwrap them one by one. White powder in the first, origami, Saskia-style. Next, a white pill, a dove logo, the obsession with flying continues. In at number three, a capsule with M printed on it, a condom for afters, and a joint rolled, ready to smoke.

I sit in the dark shadows by the wall, voices coming up the stairs towards me. I recognize Clondine's. I watch her and an older boy, the same one that grabbed Phoebe earlier, disappear into a room further down the corridor. The door to the room, left open, the sound carries. A squeal, laughter. Then silence. Five minutes or so later, a protest. Stop, no, I hear her say, stop it, Toby, I don't want to. I stick to the shadows, approach the door. Shut the fuck up, he says to her, quit crying. She won't stop, can't stop, I've been there too. Her crying distracts him, throws him off his stride, frustrated.

'Keep still, for fuck's sake.'

'Please, Toby, I don't want to.'

I push the door open, wide, the bed visible with light from a lamp in the hallway. Toby on top, Clondine pinned underneath. His knees hold her legs open, one of his hands traps her arms above her head, her jeans halfway down her thighs. Shut the fucking door, he says, a pillow thrown in my direction lands at my feet. Clondine's a baby, whimpers. I switch on the light, he turns to face me, the unwanted spectator, the killjoy. It was a bit of fun, he'd say if he was questioned, she wanted it too.

'Switch the fucking light off and disappear, pronto.'

'I heard her say no.'

'And what's that got to do with you?'

I switch the light off, a moment's reprieve for him, and me. The way Clondine is positioned on the bed reminds me. And the sound she makes, it says, don't leave me with him. I know the sound, a similar one I used to make, though mine was a she. I switch the light back on, his hand in her crotch. She lies still, like a blow-up doll. I flick the switch, a disco of sorts.

Off.

On.

Off.

On.

Offon.

Offon.

A distraction, for even the most committed rapist.

It works.

He moves off her rigid, frigid body. She rolls, a rag doll, hanging over the side of the bed, vomits. Sobs. Vomits again. Saliva and druggy sick hang off her chin. She is five years old, crumpled and used, wants her mummy. Be careful what you wish for.

He's in front of me now, my back against the door, my foot prevents it from closing.

His hand on my neck, his body against mine.

'Jealous are you? Wish it was you, do you?'

A clumsy hand between my legs, rubs crudely back and forth, friction through denim. He squeezes my breast, licks my face, I feel him hard against the waistband of my jeans. His eyes roll in his head, the drugs make him fly, doesn't he know? Superheroes don't steal, nor do they rape. Clondine whimpers again. Two against one but she's useless, out of her depth. Bite your nose off, shall I, Toby? Dream face ruined, in hiding for ever.

Like me.

I reach down, grab his dick as hard as I can. Pleasure arrives in his body from the sudden touch, but it doesn't last long as I tighten my grip, pain receptors activated. Tiny powerful neurons scream in his head. The science behind pain, a specialist topic of mine. Important to know how the process works, you said to me often, as you activated mine. I expect a black eye, a punch or a swipe, but the cat's got his tongue, or his dick. He drops to his knees on the floor. Too late to pray, Toby.

Clondine's off the bed, her hair and eyes wild and unhinged, she pulls up her jeans. Toby's down, groans on his back. A voice from the bottom of the stairs filters up to the room.

'Mate, Toby, are you up there? Come down, there's a beer bong on the go. Stevo's already spewed his load, hilarious. Dude, are you up there?'

Toby. A fish on a riverbank, a gasp here and there. His hand does not leave his dick. Sweaty and wasted, and fucked by a girl. Footsteps on the stairs, Toby moves to stand up, pride does that, it motivates. White tacky deposits gather at the sides of his mouth, a line of sweat on his upper lip. The smell of his sex cloaks around me, deep from inside his glands.

'Bitch,' he says to me.

Hugo, Huggy to his mates, arrives at the door. I walk towards Clondine.

'Dude, where the fuck have you been, I've been looking for you for ages. There's some seriously crazy shit going on in the kitchen.'

You could say the same up here.

Toby wipes his dehydrated mouth with the back of his hand, gestures towards us.

'Just having a bit of fun with the local wildlife, you know how it goes.'

'Excellent work, mate,' Huggy replies. 'But next time give me a shout, share the fun, there's a good boy.'

They leave, arms round each other's shoulders. Smug. Carefree. One with a dick that requires ice, not sympathy. I hear chanting, a game, the beer bong in full swing. Clondine sits on the edge of the bed. Legs, jelly and weak, her head in her hands. She cries, mumbles about feeling stupid.

'Don't worry,' I say. 'I won't tell Phoebe.'

She looks up at me. Make-up, black. Panda eyes. Sick in her hair. Confused.

'Why would you tell Phoebe?'

'I thought maybe she liked him, I saw him hug her when he arrived.'

'She used to but not any more, not since she met Sam. Fuck, I'm such an idiot. I've liked him for ages, I thought he liked me too.'

I offer her the elastic band from my wrist.

'You should wash your face, you can use this to put your hair up if you like.'

She's unsteady on her feet so I help her into the bathroom, I hand her a flannel I find in the cabinet under the sink. Use warm water, I tell her. It'll help.

I ask her if she needs anything else, she replies, 'Will you stay with me, just in case?'

I nod. Her words are slurred, bloodstream full of who knows what.

'I bet he tells everyone I'm a cock-tease.'

'There's a towel over there, dry your face.'

'Oh god, what a mess. I hope he doesn't come back, you don't think he will, do you?'

'No.'

'How can you be so fucking calm?'

Practice. I've had plenty.

I shrug.

'I didn't know Phoebe had a boyfriend.'

'Shit, did I tell you that? Don't tell her I told you, she doesn't want Mike to know.'

'Do you know him?'

'It's just some dude she met over the summer, he lives in Italy I think, they email each other all the time. I can't get my hands to stop shaking.'

'It's shock, it'll stop soon.'

'How do you know all this? You knew what to do when Georgie fell as well.'

'I read a lot.'

She leans into the mirror, uses a corner of the facecloth to wipe away the smudged mascara from around her eyes.

'Ugh. My mouth tastes disgusting.'

'Gargle with some mouthwash.'

'Why are you being nice to me, why did you come and help? We haven't exactly been nice to you.'

'You sounded scared.'

'I was. So stupid. Oh god, I hope he doesn't tell anyone, I'll get such a rough time at school.'

'I know what that feels like.'

She turns to face me, pupils large one minute, pinpricks the next, as she struggles to focus.

'Look, Milly, I guess I owe you a thank you about what just happened.'

'Well at least you remember my name, as in not dog-face.'

Decency to blush, a little, even when wasted.

'I guess I owe you an apology as well. I'm sorry we've been total bitches to you, it was supposed to be a laugh but it's got a bit out of hand.'

'Why me?'

'I'm not saying it was all Phoebe's fault, but most of it was her idea.'

'I don't think she likes me very much.'

'She doesn't like anybody who Mike fosters. He'd promised not to take anyone else for ages then you turn up, she's hardly going to welcome you with open arms, is she? Fuck, I think I'm going to be sick.'

She kneels on the floor, wraps her arms round the toilet, dry heaving like Clara when Georgie fell. When she stops I ask her if she needs anything.

'A new life,' she replies and laughs, swivelling her body round to face me.

If only it was as simple as that.

'Don't tell Phoebe I said this, but you know she's jealous of you, right?'

'Jealous? Of what?'

'All the time you spend with Mike.'

'It's not like that, there's just some stuff going on at the moment.'

Some pretty big stuff.

'Yeah, well, it's not like she's got her mum, is it?'

No, but let your drunken, wasted, disloyal lips tell me why. Please.

'I'd kind of noticed they weren't very close.'

'How can you be close to someone you hardly know? God, I still feel like chucking up.'

She leans her head on the toilet seat. I remove the tooth-brushes from the glass by the sink, fill it with water and hand it to her.

She nods, says thanks.

'What did you mean about Phoebe hardly knowing Saskia?'

'No way, she'd kill me if she thought I'd said anything.'

I call her bluff. I watched you do it so well with the women you looked after, how you made them think you knew more than you did. It worked every time and it works with Clondine.

'Do you mean when Saskia wasn't well?'

Clondine lifts her head, squints up at me.

'How the hell do you know?' she asks. 'Did Mike tell you?'

'Sort of, yeah.'

'Fuck. I suppose it's kind of obvious something's not right if you're living with them. She hasn't been in the mental hospital for years but probably still should be, totally lost the plot when Phoebe was born.'

I nod, as if I know what she means, and say how hard it must have been for Phoebe.

'Yeah, I think she thinks it was her fault.'

'Why?'

'I don't know. Anyway.'

'How long was she in hospital for?'

'I thought you said you knew.'

I distract her by saying her hands have stopped shaking.

She looks down at them, says, thank god, it would be the first thing her mum would've noticed, then announces she needs to pee. She hauls herself up on the toilet, pulls her jeans down. A gush of urine, a fart halfway through. Intimacy I'm only used to with you. I leave the bathroom, straighten up the bed, replace the pillow, cover the pile of sick with a magazine from the bedside table. She talks over the flush.

'I'll try and speak to Phoebs, persuade her you're not that much of a freak after all.'

She walks out of the en suite, a bit wobbly on her feet still but mainly in one piece. The ability of humans, together again on the outside, the inside, a different story. A much bigger mess.

'Can you see my other shoe?'

'It's over there by the chest of drawers.'

'Thanks. How do I look?'

'Fine.'

'Like nothing happened, hey.'

'Yeah.'

'Actually, would you mind if we don't mention to Phoebe that I was with Toby, she can be a bit possessive over the boys and I can't really be arsed with the grief.'

'Of course, but would you –'

'Lay off you at school? I'll try, sure.'

She walks to the door. I check my phone, half past eleven, thirty minutes till curfew. I make my way down shortly after her. I look for Joe, but can't see him, I find Phoebe though. A crowd around her in the kitchen, a drinking vessel in her hand. A funnel, a tube. Bong, they chant, as she drinks. Bong. Bong. Bong. I walk to the tap, fill a glass of water, happy for once their cheering and jeering isn't at me.

Wrong.

'Not so fast,' Phoebe says. 'Your turn.'

The room quietens, I ignore her. A block of knives to my left. Easy. Paint the town red, or the kitchen.

'Did you not hear me, I said it was your go.'

I turn round. She's both beautiful and wasted, pupils large and intense. Sucks on a Marlboro Light, forms an O with her lips, releases a perfect grey smoke ring. Her cheeks florid, rampant, a state of arousal. She'd have been the better candidate to go to bed with Toby.

'No thanks,' I reply.

Heckles and murmurs rise out of the crowd, we are not, but we are, in the Middle Ages still, a blood bath people would happily pay to watch. She blows a second smoke ring, so perfect I want to stick my tongue in it. The air in the room heavy, not just the smoke, but heady, her adoring fans, impatient. Oh come on, leave her be, she's not worth it. Freak. Weirdo. The usual. Then Clondine, quiet so far, says, leave her alone, she's all right. Phoebe takes a drag on her cigarette, the longest yet, turns towards her friend, exhales in her face and stubs her cigarette out on the back of Clondine's hand.

'Fuck.' She withdraws it, holds it to her chest. 'What the hell was that for?'

'Sorry, Clonny, it was an accident, I mistook you for the ashtray.'

'You're fucked in the head, you know that, seriously crazy. That was really painful.'

'Oh, stop being such a baby, here, have an ice cube.'

She takes one from a tumbler on the table, throws it in Clondine's direction, hits her on the head. Sniggers.

Clondine gathers up her bag, says, that's it, I'm done, I've had enough. I'm going home. The atmosphere in the room shifts, a departure ruins the magic, the doorway to this secret, spoilt rich kids' coven ripped off by the blast of cold air as Clondine leaves through the patio doors. A line is drawn, I see it in the room. Too far, Phoebe, you went too far. If only she was better at showing her softer side. The girl who likes to spend an evening sat on the ground by the feet of the housekeeper who brought her up. The girl who cries at night.

She stares at me, eyes full of contempt. Anger. I've seen her look at Saskia the same way.

'You're just always here, aren't you?' she says.

She points at me, eyes slanted and slurred, her knees buckle a little. I turn to face the sink again. One by one, excuses are made, vague talk about tidying up.

'Don't worry, the olds are away until Monday. I'll pay Ludy extra, she'll sort it out tomorrow,' I hear Matty say.

'Good old Ludy,' someone jokes.

In the reflection of the window I see Toby drape himself round Phoebe. I should ask him how his dick is, rape boy. She shrugs him off, walks through to the living room. He follows, 'Let me take you home.'

'Whatever.'

I should warn her he's not a great chaperone. I bet he produces a key for one of the private gardens on the way — either that or gives her a leg up, tosses her over. The last few people leave the kitchen. I notice Phoebe's handbag on the counter, hear her laughing with the hyena girl from earlier. On my way past I tell her it's almost midnight but she ignores me so I leave on my own.

Mike lets me in when I arrive, he must have been waiting by the window, anxious.

'Where's Phoebe?' he asks.

'Just coming I think, she's walking with one of the boys.'

'Oh god, that phase in life already,' he says with a smile. Asks me if I had a good time.

'Not bad, I'm pretty zonked though. Can I have my pill, then I'm off to bed.'

'Sure.'

Two hours pass, curfew been and gone. I wonder how long it took her to realize her house keys were missing, slipped into my pocket as I passed her bag. She and her enlarged pupils will have to face the music.

Eventually I hear footsteps coming up the stairs, muffled voices, something about dealing with this in the morning. The door along from mine closes with a slam. I fall asleep immediately, content in the knowledge.

That round was mine.

21

The sensation of falling jerks me awake. I thought I was in court and I couldn't remember how to answer the questions. Everybody was staring at me, waiting. You, behind the screen. I get out of bed, go into the bathroom, update the number in charcoal, the countdown I've been keeping, change it to eight, lean my head against the cabinet door and try to breathe.

Bare feet are silent, Mike doesn't notice me standing in the kitchen doorway. He's reading something, holds a page in the air as he looks at the one underneath. I can't be sure but I think I see my name at the top. He underlines, annotates as he reads, rubs his eyes, harassed, tired. I can't but I want to, walk over and hug him. Thank him for having me. For caring.

He looks up, turns the paper over as I approach the table, slides the pages under his diary. I make a mental note to look for them later, or perhaps on a Thursday when Saskia's at yoga and Mike stays late at work.

'I didn't notice you standing there. Would you like some breakfast?' he asks.

'Maybe in a bit. I might make some tea. Would you like some, you look tired?'

'I waited up for Phoebe. Not only was she two hours late but she managed to lose her keys at some point.'

Oh.

'Sorry, I did try to get her to leave with me.'

'Don't apologize, it's not your fault, at least one of you made it home on time.'

'Shall I make Saskia a cup as well?'

'That's very sweet but she's actually up and out already, she and the girls headed off early to some kind of outlet, a big designer sale apparently.'

While the kettle boils he asks me if I'm looking forward to going away tomorrow. I nod, tell him that after he told me we were going to Tetbury, I looked it up online.

'Did you find the Arboretum? It's very close to there, it's called Westonbirt. I think you'll like it, there's lots of nice walks. We used to take Phoebe when she was little.'

He used to, he means. Saskia there maybe, but not really. I don't need to ask how he takes his tea, I enjoy how at home that makes me feel.

'Once you're done, Milly, come and sit down, there's something I need to talk to you about.'

The teabags have stewed enough, the water surrounding them a deep brown, but I push them under, drown them, delay joining him at the table. I add milk to both, one sugar for me, none for him, stir, then take the mugs over, sit down opposite him. I tuck my legs into my chest, feet off the ground, the monsters that lurk, grab you. Don't let go.

'Thanks,' he says, moving his chair closer into the table. 'I don't want you to take this the wrong way, you've got an awful lot on your plate right now, but I think it's important to talk about the email Ms James sent me.'

About MK.

The tea is too hot, I take a large gulp anyway. Tongue. Burnt.

'Ms James mentioned you'd given Miss Kemp a present, a candle, and that you'd been seeing her quite a bit.'

'Not that much, no.'

'Perhaps a bit more than other pupils might see their guidance teachers?'

'Only so she can help me with my art.'

'I know, but you've also been emailing her a lot I believe.'

'Only a few times. She hadn't replied, I wanted to make sure she was getting them.'

'A few times a week is quite a lot, Milly. I'm sure Miss Kemp likes you very much but she's been feeling a bit overwhelmed. I think perhaps you'd like to spend more time with her than she can manage.'

I feel humiliated and stupid and overcome with desire for you. It didn't happen often, you weren't often in a good mood, but occasionally you'd stand behind me brushing my hair. You told me how pretty I was and I felt it too. I always felt prettier when you did nice things.

'I can see how the confusion might have occurred. I've met Miss Kemp a number of times, she's a lovely woman, very kind. But I think it's important to help you label and understand what might be going on. Do you have any idea what I mean?'

'No.'

'Have you heard of a term called transference?'

I say no again, but it's not true, I've read about it in one of his books. He's wrong though, that's not what's happening with MK. I enjoy her company, that's all.

Isn't it?

'Transference is a process by which someone unconsciously transfers feelings about a person in their past on to a person or situation in their present.'

'I was only trying to thank her.'

Not ask her to be my mum.

'And it was a very thoughtful gesture but it would have been okay, better even, if you'd just said it to her.'

I bite down on my tongue, the pain, and having to stifle a reaction, sends a sharp twinge through the lower part of my spine, the way the nerves are connected inside a body.

'Nobody's blaming you, Milly, it's a very normal feeling for you to have.'

There it is, the difference, flagged up about me again.

A normal feeling for 'you' to have.

Mike's face swims around in front of me, tears, rogue joy-riders, land on my knees. He tells me it's okay, not to punish myself for having these feelings.

'Does it mean I can't see her any more?'

'We've agreed you can work with her on your portfolio for the art prize until the end of term. After that we'll see, none of us know what'll be happening then anyway.'

To me, he means.

In the sanctuary of my room I take out my sketches. Portraits of you. A gallery of the darkest parts of my mind, where you live. I tell you I'm sorry about MK, it won't happen again. I hear a message come through on my phone, walk over to the bed, read it. It's Morgan, confirming we're still meeting at the bottom of the garden at six. Yes, I reply, hearing Phoebe in the corridor, shouting:

'I don't care!'

'Well you should,' Mike responds.

I listen through the door.

'Why should I stay at home, you're never around anyway.'

'That's not the point,' Mike replies.

'I DON'T FUCKING CARE. LEAVE ME ALONE.'

I lean into the wood. Child and parent, no other relation-ship more complicated exists. Her bedroom door slams shut, I move away from mine, put the sketches back into the drawer under my bed and sit down at my desk, try and do some homework, but I'm too angry and ashamed by how wrong I got it with MK. You never got it wrong, you knew how to be with everybody. The women's faces would light up as you walked into work, the children's too. I used to watch you, hoping one day I could be that version of you.

When it's time to meet Morgan I'm unsure if I should go, I recognize the feelings inside. A dark colour. Not good. I wouldn't have gone if she hadn't called me saying she was already there. Waiting. Hurry up, she said, it's freezing. I put on a jumper and leave my room using the fire stairs attached to my balcony, stay flat against the perimeter wall of the garden, the security light only activated if you cross on to the gravel or grass. I know, I've tested it. She's in the bottom corner next to the gate leading to the close. It's dark by six o'clock now and as my eyes adjust I can see the details of her face, and that she's eating a sandwich.

'It's got crisps in it,' she says. 'Remember you gave me a packet when we first met?'

I nod.

'So, what's been happening?'

'Nothing much, just some stuff at school.'

'What kind of stuff?'

'To do with one of the teachers.'

'Eww, like a creepy teacher?'

It turns out I'm the creep.

'No, just a misunderstanding.'

'Did he try and touch you or something?'

'It's a she, not a he.'

'Even worse.'

Yes, the public feel that way about you too. A woman

killing children. Newspapers opened at breakfast tables, milk in stripy jugs curdled all around the world when it was first reported. Cereal spat out of mouths. I kick the wall with my foot. Hot molten lava bleeds inside me.

'What's up with you, I was only joking.'

I tell her nothing's wrong but what I should say is: stay away, I don't feel like me. Or maybe this is me, this is who I am, someone standing in front of a friend fighting the urge to do something, to cause pain so it's shared, so it's not just me.

She eats noisily. The crunching of the crisps, the sound pollutes the silence I need. Usually her company helps but not today. I keep thinking about the lawyers, their questions. What did you see on the night Daniel died? What happened? I saw my mother. You saw her do what?

'Is it about your mum, is that why you're stressed out? I saw something on the news by the way, it said she was a nurse. Fucking crazy, imagine being looked after by her.'

'I don't want to talk about it, Morgan, stop it.'

'It might help if you talk about it, it's not your fault she's mental. It also said she had a kid living at home with her – if it wasn't you, who was it? I never knew you had any brothers or sisters.'

'I don't.'

None that I want to talk about.

'Who do you reckon it was at home with her then?'

I shrug. 'I've asked you already, Morgan, please stop.'

Silence is better, say nothing at all. Please. Too many questions. Too many voices filling up my head. THAT'S NOT TRUE, ANNIE, IT'S ONLY MINE. The lava inside me scorches anything good or gentle along the way. I watch Morgan's mouth move, the way she licks her lips. Eat them, eat it all up. I want her to stop talking about you.

'My lot reckon she'll go down for life, you'll never see her again, which is probably just as well.'

'Shut up, Morgan, I mean it. That's the last time I'm going to tell you.'

'Jesus, talk about being sensitive, she's a fucking monster, you should be glad I hate her.'

Eats like an animal, all over her face. Her teeth and her tongue. Still talking about you, isn't she. YES SHE IS, WHAT ARE YOU GOING TO DO? Good wolf. Bad wolf. Crunch. Crisps. Tongue. Lips. I move to diffuse the bad, tell her I'm cold, I'm going inside.

'Why are you so angry? You don't care about her, do you?'

Couldn't put Humpty together again.

The sandwich gets it first, smacked out of her hand, her arm next. I pin her against the wall, the place we arranged to meet no longer feels safe. I use my height, squeeze her arm with my fingers, think about what shape and colour the bruise will be.

'Get off,' she says. 'Stop it.'

It used to be me who said that, the tables now turned, the shoe on the other foot. It feels good to be bad. I'm sorry, I can't help it, but she's no longer talking about you so maybe being bad sometimes works. I might have done something worse but when she says, maybe you're more like your mother than you think, the hot lava recedes, turns purple. Cools. Sick. A sickness inside me. I let go of her arm, step back, lean over. My hands on my thighs. Can't be. Like you. Don't want to be.

Neither of us speaks, processing it in our own ways. I turn to face her, she rubs her hand up and down her arm.

'Morgan, I'm sorry. I don't know what happened.'

'Yeah, well, it won't be happening again.'

'What do you mean?'

'You can get to fuck, that's what I mean.'

I try to hug her but she uses her arms to block me, pushes me back and leaves. I sit on the ground for a while, look up at the winter sky, only one star. I look away and when I look back it's gone.

It doesn't want me to see it.

I sing while I look for them.

Eight green bottles, hanging on the wall. No. Not bottles, something else, and not on the wall. I try the song again, your words instead.

There are eight little somethings hidden in the cellar, I thought there was nine, but the ninth didn't make it down there. Remember?

Yes.

If I could just open the door I could check the little somethings are okay.

Can't open. The door.

'Milly, it's Saskia. The door's locked, Mike locked it, what are you singing?'

And if one little something should accidentally fall. Can't open. The door.

'I'm getting Mike.'

Can you hear me, little somethings? I've come to let you out. But they don't reply, it's too late. I'm too late.

They've already fallen.

Which means they'll have to stay.

22

I'm woken by the sound of Phoebe leaving for the hockey tour to Cornwall, voices in the corridor, a door opening and closing. Monday. I should get up, we're going away, but my body feels heavy, weighed down by the shame of what I did to Morgan.

By the volume of your voice.

When Saskia knocks on my door, asks if she can come in, I say yes and sit up in bed.

White jeans, skinny, tight. A baby blue and white striped shirt tucked in, the top half of her hair pushed forward in a bump, secured with a brown hair clip with teeth, the rest hanging long over her shoulders.

'I hope I didn't wake you, we wanted to let you sleep in after.'

After last night.

'We're going to leave soon. The drive should only take about an hour and a half, we'll be there by lunch.'

She doesn't say anything else about last night. Mike will have told her not to, explained to expect this in the run-up to the trial.

'Milly.'

'Sorry, I was –'

'A million miles away?'

Further.

'Something like that, yeah.'

She fiddles with her necklace, brings it up, presses the points of the letters to her lips. The flesh turns white where it's pressed, turns pink again. She asks me if I need help packing.

'No thank you, I'll be down shortly.'

When she closes the door I reach for my phone to see if Morgan's replied, but she hasn't. I battle with anxiety as I wash my face, get dressed and pack an overnight bag. What I did to Morgan was wrong and I don't want to lose her as a friend, but I'm also worried she might tell people about me. About who I am.

When I get downstairs, Rosie's in the hallway next to Mike and Saskia's holdalls. She wags her tail when she sees me. I put my bag down, rub between her ears.

'I don't think you're coming,' I tell her. 'You're staying here with Sevita. Next time maybe.'

She cocks her head, licks my hand and pads into the kitchen alongside me.

'There's freshly squeezed orange juice over there, would you like some?' Saskia offers.

'No thanks, I'm going to make some toast.'

Mike's on his mobile facing away from us, leaning into the sink.

'Of course, I'll bring her Wednesday after we get back, does that work for you? Okay, sure. Thanks, June, see you then.'

He hangs up, turns round to face us.

'That was June, we've arranged for you to go in and watch your video evidence this Wednesday, three o'clock. I'll take you.'

I nod, appetite gone.

*

The traffic is slow leaving London but a long stretch of motorway follows, the roadsides greener as we get further away from the city. Mike asks me how my sketches are coming along for the art prize. Fine, I tell him. Saskia turns and says she'd love to see them some time. She and Mike exchange a smile and she places her hand on the back of his neck for a moment. It's the first time I've seen her touch him.

After an hour or so we turn into a long gravel driveway, a fountain in the middle when we reach the end. A member of staff explains to Mike that the car park's full, what with it being half-term and all.

'Leave the key in the ignition, we'll move it into an overspill in the field over there. Hang on to this ticket and whenever you need the car show it to reception and they'll arrange for it to be brought round for you.'

Mike checks us in and we're shown to our rooms, a family suite, separate bedrooms with an adjoining door. When we go down for lunch I'm struck by how many children there are. Crawling; running; crying; spilling. Everywhere. But it's not just children, you're here too. Your face, on the front of a newspaper, the headline 'One Week to Go'. A man at a table by the window, he holds you. Reads you. Folds you. Places you in the inside pocket of the coat handed to him by one of the waitresses. He stands up and puts it on. How close your face lies to his heart. But truth be told, you love in a different way from most. Your love isn't so gentle and kind to be a kiss from your lips to a person's heart. It isn't like that at all.

Mike asks if I'm okay. Yes, I'm fine, I tell him. I don't want to ruin the trip by letting him know you came too.

After lunch we spend the afternoon walking in the grounds, stop and have a few conversations with other families. Mike bumps into somebody he works with. The man kisses Saskia and when I'm introduced, he says, 'So this is Milly.'

Mike nods and smiles, yes. Yes it is. The man explains that Cassie, his wife, is here too but she's gone to change the baby.

'And these little scruff pots are also mine.'

Two small boys, no older than five or six, play chase in and out of his legs. It looks fun, I wouldn't mind joining in. Simple game. No harm. Later on in the afternoon children's activities are set up on the front lawn, a bit like a school sports day. Saskia and me sit in the armchairs by the window, watch them. Ring o' roses, the egg and spoon, even a race for the dads, not for the mums though, if there was and you were here in flesh and blood, you'd have joined in, you'd probably have won. Mike arrives, yawns, suggests we all have an early night. He explained to me during our walk in the afternoon that he locked the door to the cellar last week, didn't want me to hurt myself. I thanked him, wished I could tell him not being able to check what's down there hurts me more.

After dinner we go to our separate rooms. A reply from Morgan, two words only.

Fuck you.

The next morning over breakfast we decide to take the car to the Arboretum. The sky is overcast, rain threatens. Mike says not to worry, Phoebe's wellies and waterproof jacket are in the car, we brought them for you.

'Won't she mind?' I ask.

'We won't tell her if you don't,' replies Saskia, with an unusually playful look on her face. All three of us smile.

We head to our rooms to brush our teeth, arrange to meet in reception ten minutes later. The man we spoke to yesterday, John, is there when I arrive, by the front desk, with a woman I presume is Cassie, his wife, and the two boys, along with a baby she holds in her arms. Cassie and Saskia have never met, comment politely on how chilly it is, a perfect day for an open fire.

'I think there's one in the front lounge,' Saskia says.

Cassie suggests we have coffee there before we head out. Once we're seated Mike and John engage in a conversation about the refurb of their office. John complains that the waiting room lacks privacy, can be seen from the street.

'Yes, not ideal, perhaps we should look at blinds or some kind of screen,' Mike replies.

The word: screen. Like the one that'll be in court next week separating you and me.

The two older children sit on the floor by the French windows, to the right of the fireplace. A basket of toys which they proceed to tip over, cries of *brum-brum* as they play with cars, an attempt at a gunshot noise when one of them finds a plastic water pistol. A small slice of winter sun creeps in, breaks through the layer of clouds in the sky, lands perfectly around the boys, the gold of their hair, the blue of their eyes. Little angels. Again, I'm drawn to join in, or cry, so beautiful. In the end I do nothing, stay where I am, not sure either crying or joining in would be welcome, or normal. When I turn back, Mike's watching me, a strange look on his face, attempts to smile when he sees me noticing. Cassie begins a conversation with Saskia about Wetherbridge.

'Obviously it's years away,' she says, looking down at the

baby girl in her arms. 'But it's always good to hear an insider's view.'

Saskia's transfixed by the baby, shifts her gaze but it ends up back there. Cassie notices, asks if she'd like to hold her.

'No thanks, I'm not very good with babies.'

'What about you, would you like to?' she asks me.

'Yes please.'

The words fly out of my mouth, she stands up, transfers the baby into my arms. Flushed skin, her eyes closed, a sweet curtain of lashes so long they almost touch the upper part of her cheeks. There's nothing in her mouth, no dummy or bottle, but she makes a continual sucking movement with her perfectly peach lips, in and then out. A small flower bud.

Beautiful, pure things make me feel ugly. Tarnished. I remember asking you when I was three, maybe four, where I came from. I waited for you to sweep me up, rub our noses together in an Eskimo kiss and reply, you came from me, you belong with me, I love you. Just like the mummy of another little girl did when I saw her ask the same question at school, but you didn't respond, walked out of the kitchen, left me standing there alone.

Cassie says to Mike, your daughter's a natural, and just for a moment, a split second, I feel what it's like to be mistaken for theirs.

'Actually, Milly's our foster daughter, Phoebe's on a hockey trip,' Mike replies.

'I told you that last night, Cassie,' John adds.

'Sorry, baby brain. That's great though, I really admire you guys for taking on –'

Someone like me.

She doesn't get to finish her sentence, the baby lets out a

loud angry wail. Eyes open, looking at me. Scared. She sensed it. Whatever it is inside of me. Felt me holding her that little bit too tightly. Even tighter when Mike said I wasn't their daughter. I hand her back to her mother, safe hands. You'd hope so.

We drive to the Arboretum and when we arrive it's busy. Couples, families, the occasional person on their own. Exotic shrubs and painstakingly manicured tree-lined avenues, the autumnal colours, burnt oranges and yellows, an intense crimson echo from the red leaves on the trees above. We walk mainly in silence. I think it means we're comfortable, a nice thought. Happy. Mike comments that there aren't many kids my age here.

'I'm afraid it's not so cool to holiday with parents any more.'

'It doesn't matter,' I reply. 'I'm enjoying that it's just the three of us.'

Mike smiles, relaxed. And though he would never admit it out loud, I know he agrees, a sense of relief at not having to be the go-between for Saskia and Phoebe. Nicer all round.

Later that evening after dinner I buy Morgan a snow globe from the hotel gift shop. Fir trees, two children holding hands, a snowman built next to them. I text her again, tell her I've bought her a present. No reply.

At first I think I'm imagining it, or it's the TV through the wall, but as I move closer to the adjoining door, place my ear flat against it, I hear them. Arguing. Saskia was drunk at dinner, virtually mute apart from hiccups following dessert which of course she was too full to eat. Mike says something about her getting a grip, especially with the court case next week. I'm trying, she says. Try harder, he replies. Something's thrown, a glass maybe, it hits the wall. Their voices lower, she begins to cry. I imagine Mike holding her, telling her it's okay. After a while their voices stop, other noises instead. The moaning from Saskia makes me feel funny. Involved. When the noises stop I take off my clothes, run my fingers up and down the white scar ladders on both sides of my ribs, then climb into the shower.

Scrub my skin raw.

23

Five days to go.

I walk over to the balcony door, open the curtains, a robin is there on the railing. Its breast, red. Puffed out in the cold. When it sees me, it flies off. Doesn't feel safe any more. I don't blame it.

When we got back from the Cotswolds on Wednesday I went to the court with Mike to review my video evidence. It wasn't easy to watch. The girl on the screen talking about her mother. That girl was me.

I wish I could retract my statement, be able to say:

That didn't happen.

But it did.

While I was there the lawyers took me through a mock cross-examination.

Did you know Daniel Carrington?

Yes.

How did you know him?

He was one of the children at my mother's work.

Were you in the house when she brought him home?

Yes.

The lawyers warned me the defence will do anything, and everything, to trip me up, make me look like an unreliable witness. How do you feel about that, Fatty asked. I said I felt fine.

I lied.

June showed me the courtroom, the stand I'd be on and

where the screen to shield me from you would be. The reality of being close to you again produced a Pavlovian response, excess saliva in my mouth, so much so, I thought I'd be sick. The trial starts on Monday but I've been told now that I'll be presenting on the Thursday and Friday. I had to change the number in the bathroom cabinet – the countdown was never for the trial, but for when I'd get to be with you.

It's Bonfire Night tonight. Mike told me if I watched from my balcony I'd see the fireworks display a family a few streets along from us have in their garden every year. It usually starts around seven, he said. Morgan still hasn't been in touch so I text her again, tell her about it, invite her over. I can sneak you in, I write.

Mike and I met yesterday to focus on breathing. What to do if I feel panicky on the stand. He asked me if there was anything I was unsure of, anything I wanted to go over again before I faced the defence next week. No, I don't think so, I told him, what happened is clear in my mind. He asked me to think of a word that made me feel good. It took me a while but in the end I chose freedom. I told him I envied you, out in the open, whereas I live in the dark, hidden from all but a few. Everything taken from me, even my name. He told me to view the darkness as a place to rest; in the future it'll become light. What if I'm like her, I asked him, what if I inherit it? *Monoamine oxidase A*. The enzyme for violence. If it's in her, it's likely it's in me, but he told me I'm nothing like you, he knows that for sure. I'm not certain I believe he meant it, or if he believes it himself.

I didn't forget about the morning in the kitchen when I saw him hide the notes from me so when he and Saskia were both out on Thursday, I went into his study. It didn't take long to find them, the bottom-left drawer, under a textbook.

The heading on the first page: **MILLY (ideas for book)**.

I only managed to photocopy half of them, the front door opening and closing, Sevita coming in. She smiled when she saw me in the hallway, the originals back where I found them, the copies tucked neatly into the waistband of my jeans. It turns out Mike's writing a book about me, about how I'm surviving, him at my side. He refers to the dream I told him I'd had. You, trapped in a burning room. When he asked me what happened in the dream I told him the truth. I rescued you. Every single time, I rescued you. Written in red pen below, 'still shows great loyalty to mum, discuss guilt'.

Some of his other footnotes detail my self-blame, how a victim of abuse loses the perspective of neutrality — everybody for or against them. An arrow in red, then the phrase 'GOOD ME vs BAD ME', underlined and circled.

I've been trying to work out how I feel about Mike writing a book about me. He hasn't asked my permission, I never signed a form. Am I his project? A meal ticket to fame in his profession. A success story. He thinks. He hopes. If it means I get to stay here longer, I don't mind. Access to my mind is a currency I'm willing to pay.

I see Saskia at lunchtime, ask her if she's missing Phoebe, who's still away on tour. She smiles, says, of course, I miss both her and Mike when they're away, it's nice having you here. Her body language, the way she shifts from one foot to the other, the way she fiddles with her hair, tells me another story. It tells me that when it's just me and her, she's uncomfortable still. On edge.

I spend the rest of the day reading about you. The news websites, you're top of the bill. A reporter outside the courthouse running through what'll happen when the trial starts. He reels off your crimes, the number nine used three times. Nine children. Nine bodies. Nine charges of murder.

By the time I've read everything I can find, it's getting dark outside, not long until the fireworks. I go to the toilet and when I come out of the bathroom I see movement on the balcony. The robin's not back, but Morgan is.

I close my laptop, unlock the door, my heart keen in my chest. Her hood pulled up, covering most of her face.

'I'm sorry, Morgan. I really, really am.'

She shrugs, looks down at her feet. I reach for her hand, bring her inside, show her the snow globe.

'Shake it.'

And when she does, I know we're going to be okay.

Forgiving, that's what she is, and lonely. A person can forgive a lot if they need the company.

When the fireworks start we go on to the balcony. Brightly coloured rockets and explosions paint the sky.

'Don't ever do anything like that again,' she says, after the display finishes. 'You hurt me.'

'I know, and I won't. Did you tell anybody about it?'

She shakes her head, looks disappointed I asked that, then leaves, taking the snow globe with her.

I hear you coming, weaving your way across the thick carpet in my bedroom.

You've got a message for me, something you'd like to say. SEE YOU IN COURT, ANNIE.

Up eight. Up another four.
The door on the right.

You wanted to cut off my hair, long down my back, to short as a boy's.

But you didn't, it would draw attention to me at school.

You still had your fun though.

Dressed me up, stuffed my knickers with socks.

But I wasn't enough for you.

The room in our house that had lain empty for months.

The room opposite mine.

You announced it to me at dinner one night.

The playground, that's what I'll call it, you said.

Insatiable.

I knew you'd never be through, so I took my chance to leave you too.

24

Day one of your trial. I say no when Mike suggests I stay off school for the week. He's trying to shield me. The press. Erupted. Every news report and headline I read online before breakfast, fill to overflowing with you. The BBC website shows the crowd gathering outside the courthouse. A mob. Angry. If they could they'd hammer on the van as you pass. Spit on it. Throw paint bombs, the colour of red. Murderer. Murderer.

The silence in the house is deafening, the radio in the kitchen unplugged. Mike jokes to us all, I think we should try and do a week, maybe two, without TV. Phoebe says she doesn't care, she'll watch Netflix on her laptop. This morning before I leave the house Mike pulls me to one side, tells me to come home straight away if school gets too much. What about if it all gets too much, I wanted to ask.

If I'd thought about it, been clever about it, I'd have stayed at home, missed swimming this morning. Stupid. Head, foggy. I change in a cubicle, thankful the scars and cuts on my ribs are hidden by where my costume sits. I'd tell them if I could, that I open my skin to bleed out the bad, let the good in. But they wouldn't get it, they'd ask, what are you talking about, what bad?

A line of canoes faces us, rescue training essential for the Duke of Edinburgh scheme. We're split into groups of four, whoever we're standing next to. I should have paid more attention.

'Come on, girls,' Mrs Havel says, hurrying us up. 'Has everybody got a group to work with? Wonderful. Line up at the edge of the pool.'

Clondine tries to be nice.

'Oh, come on, Phoebs, she's not that bad.'

Challenged in public, by one of her own. She tells Clondine, 'Shut up, you don't even know her.'

She's right.

'No, but I know you,' Clondine responds, flashing the healing cigarette burn on the back of her hand.

We're at the opposite end of the pool from the instructor. Hushed whispers pass back and forth, loud enough for me to hear. Phoebe and Izzy comment on the way my swimsuit fits, how dark the hair on my arms is. An old scar interests them, purple and large, on my right forearm.

'Bet you she did it herself.'

'Yeah, bet she did, probably into S and M.'

An eruption of giggles.

'Quieten down, you girls at the end.'

The purple crater in my arm. No. I didn't do it myself, that's not how it happened. You said as you did it, Mummy, it's so you'll never forget. A branding. You held my arm against the heated towel rail in our bathroom. You'll always be mine, you said. A tattoo of our love scorched into my arm.

The instructor enters the pool, demonstrates how to roll in a canoe. The difference between life and death, he says, when he comes back up from the blue. Relax. Trust in the water, and your partner too. Whatever you do, don't panic.

I watch him, his mouth moves yet the sound is distorted. Slow motion. It takes me a moment to realize I'm falling. Shoved into the pool. Whispers first, something like, just do it, push her, go on. I land in the water with force, the tiles on the bottom bruising my legs. I use them as purchase to swim up for air. A row of heads all in a line stare at me as I surface. Girl soldiers in black Lycra, arms not at their sides but folded over their developing breasts. Laughter, a round of applause breaks.

I swim to the edge, the instructor makes a joke about a keen bean. Phoebe offers me her hand as I approach the poolside. I know what she plans, I can see inside her mind and it doesn't look dissimilar to mine. I take her hand, one foot up on the side of the pool, halfway out, then she lets go. This time I land flat on my back, the impact of the water stings my skin. More whoops and laughter.

'Oh, for heaven's sake, Phoebe, grow up, that was stupid and dangerous, not to mention time-wasting for the rest of the class. I suggest you and Milly partner up for the canoe roll, see if you can be all sensible together, and for pete's sake, Milly, hurry up, or do I have to get a rod and fish you out?'

'No, Mrs Havel.'

I swim to the steps, satisfied by the look on Phoebe's face. The joke's on you now, canoe partner.

'Actually, Mrs Havel, I could use a volunteer and as you're already in the water —' The instructor points at me.

'Excellent idea, swim this way please, Milly.'

When I get to him he asks me to climb into the canoe while he holds it still. It's all about communication he says, and trust.

'Ready?'

I nod, gripping tight on to the sides.

'Rolling on three, okay? One, two, three, and under.'

A blur of blue, up in a flash.

'How was that?'

'It was okay.'

'See, girls, a piece of cake. If you split into pairs for this next bit please, those without canoes can practise assisted swimming. Simply get your partner to lie on their backs in the water pretending to be unconscious. It's your job to swim them to the side, keeping their nose and mouth clear of the water at all times.'

'Mrs Havel, can't I work with Izzy or Clondine?'

'No, you and Milly will work together. If you hadn't been so keen to muck around earlier you might have had the luxury of choice, but not now. Your turn for the roll.'

The noise in the pool, splashes and screams, a nervousness in the air, nobody likes the idea of rolling under water. Marie complains about chlorine, the damage to her hair. I swim over to Phoebe, hold the canoe still. Her turn to roll. Perhaps she sees inside parts of my mind too, the thoughts I'm having, because she says, 'Don't try anything funny, okay?'

My silence unnerves her, works every time.

'I mean it, otherwise you'll pay.'

I nod, fingers crossed behind my back.

While she's climbing in I'm tempted to ask her about Sam. Her laptop, left behind in her room over half-term. I was surprised, yet pleased, to find it could be accessed with no password. Setting a password was the first thing I did when I was given mine. No need, she thinks. Mike's the sort of parent who would never look without asking first. A firm believer in respecting privacy, in letting us be teenagers.

I check behind me. The instructor is busy. Mrs Havel, at the other end of the pool. Girls being girls, absorbed in themselves. I tell Phoebe I'll count to three, then roll.

'Just hurry the fuck up,' she says.

So I do. One, two, three and roll, all the way over.

Not.

Quite.

I stop halfway through. One elephant. Two elephant.

Three.

She realizes at three. Her hands uncross from her chest, thump on the sides of the canoe. I feel her body move, whacking and writhing from side to side.

Six elephant.

Seven.

The noise in the pool bounces off the tiles, laughter and coughing as water is cleared from mouths. Nobody looks, nobody notices. How long can the average person hold their breath underwater? Thirty seconds? Sixty?

Nine elephant.

Ten.

Her nails dig into my hand, a vague swirl of pink in the water. Half-moon-shaped injuries, carved out by beautifully filed nails, her pride and joy. The instructor moves closer, Mrs Havel too. I roll the canoe, her head is up, out of the water. Emotions. A rainbow of colour across her face. Panic. Fear follows next. Relief she's alive, and fury, the last to make an appearance. I revel in every single shade. She gasps, her chest heaves up and down, looks at me.

'You bitch,' she says. 'Mrs Havel. Miss.'

The instructor blows his whistle, shouts for us to switch over, those who've done the canoe roll now practise rescue swimming, and vice versa.

'Mrs Havel.'

'For goodness' sake, Phoebe, can't it wait?'

Clondine and Izzy swim towards us, it's Phoebe's face

they see. Pale. Panic. Stuck on repeat. The feeling her lungs are about to burst. Trapped.

'What's wrong?' Izzy asks.

'I almost fucking drowned, that's what's wrong,' she replies, staring at me. The whites of her eyes slightly red, the chlorine.

'Drama queen,' Izzy teases.

'Fuck off, Iz, all of you just fuck off.'

She climbs out of the canoe, swims to the steps nearest Mrs Havel and hauls herself out of the water. Goosebumps visible on her skin. You get them when you're cold, other reasons too. Her hand reaches to her throat, reassuring herself she can breathe. I don't know what she says to Mrs Havel but whatever it is she's allowed to leave the pool and doesn't return for the last part of the lesson.

In her emails to Sam she mentioned me – there's something I don't like about her, she wrote. In what way, he asked. Don't know, she's just a bit of a weirdo or something.

Or something, Phoebe.

At the end of the lesson as I swim the canoe back up to the shallows, my right hand nips. Four indentations, the shape of her fear. Behind the privacy of the cubicle door I use my phone to photograph my hand. A keepsake.

25

The following day at school I remained on high alert, knowing Phoebe wouldn't wait long to get me back. Tit for tat. A game of cat and mouse. A matter of time.

I wasn't supposed to but I also went to see MK, and as I walked up to her room I was aware of my eyes. Dry. Click as I blink, not enough sleep, a thought that unnerves me knowing I'll be on the stand in two days. I don't know what's happening in court, Mike said he and June were in touch daily but I should focus on myself, on getting as much sleep as possible before Thursday. I'd like that too but every time I close my eyes, I see nine little somethings, crying, pointing at me, asking for help.

I told MK what Mike and I agreed, that I'd be off school Thursday and Friday for a small procedure. 'Nothing serious, I hope?' she asked.

No, only the severing of an umbilical cord.

Should've been removed years ago. Toxic.

As I get undressed to shower before bed, I keep hearing your voice, imagining you standing, waiting for me outside the courtroom tossing a coin. Heads or tails. The elongated one you had made when we visited a seaside town in Wales last year, not for a holiday, new territory you wanted to explore, you said. New hunting ground, is what you meant. When I went to the toilet you asked the man at the stall to stamp both sides of the coin with the same. Heads we play, tails we don't, you said when we got home. It took me months to work out, both sides were heads. You won, every time. But you're not the judge any more, a man in a wig is. Twelve other people too. You don't get to decide this time. They do.

I didn't even hear her open the bathroom door, too busy lathering shampoo on my head, trying to quieten your voice. She yanks the shower curtain to one side. Enough time to cover my ribs with my arms, hide the scars, but not my breasts or my crotch. The flash on her phone, she takes what she needs.

'That'll teach you to try and drown me, bitch.'

I wrap the shower curtain around me, scared she'll pull it down, but she doesn't. She asks me if I've been anywhere interesting lately. When I don't reply, she says, 'Don't think I don't know all about your little friend from the estate.'

Hide. Don't show. Steam making it hard to breath. Hot.

'I'm right, aren't I? Izzy said she saw you with the little shit that sits outside the house. What's the matter, can't find friends your own age? Maybe I'll tell Dad and he can ask you about it in your "private" time. Wonder what he'd think if he knew you were hanging out with one of the estate rats, especially one much younger.'

She's twelve, almost thirteen. Small for her age. And I know what your dad would think. He'd be worried.

'Pathetic. That's what you are. I bet you loved it in the Cotswolds without me, playing happy families with my parents.'

I did, yes.

'Not that I care, it won't be long until you're gone any-way, you probably won't even get to stay for Christmas.'

I look at her angry face. I should reach out, offer her my hand and say, let's shake on it. Call a truce. Let's do this together, think of the fun we could have. Think of the mischief. But the temptation to push back, to fight, is so much stronger. Her fault, she keeps feeding the wrong wolf, giving it permission to be in charge. So instead of trying to make peace, I say to her, 'I hear you at night sometimes.'

'What? What are you talking about?'

'I hear you.'

A bullseye on her body, square in her chest, stops her in her tracks. She knows what I mean, that I hear her cry. I might be naked but she's just been laid out bare.

It takes only minutes after she leaves for my phone to vibrate, she'll have got my new number from the blackboard by the front door, Mike insists everybody's is up there. I unfold myself from the shower curtain, wrap a towel round me, walk over to my desk and pick up my phone. A picture message. Hair frothy with shampoo, skin shiny, arms folded round my ribs. Nipples hard, a dark bush below.

I can see she sent it to a number of people. Girls and boys, Joe included maybe. I walk back into the bathroom, drop my towel. Slice. Once. Twice. Red. A more interesting photo, if only she'd asked.

26

Before I left for school this morning Saskia gave me a small velvet pouch. It's a present, she said, from the crystal shop on Portobello Road. When I opened it, took it out, rolled it around my palm, the edges rough and raw, the top and bottom smooth and black, she told me it was a Black Tourmaline. The talisman of protection. I thought you could keep it in your pocket while you're in court, I thought it might help, she said. I thanked her but the gesture, although kind, made me feel worse, reminded me I needed protection.

I don't feel ready for tomorrow, a dark-coloured bruise. Aubergine. Indigo. Deep inside. Pulsates. I go over the lawyers' questions in my head as I walk to school – tell the court what your mother did, tell the court what you saw – but I can't remember the answers.

Just tell the truth, Mike says.

Easier said.

We meet in the hall for a run-through of the play. The words, their meaning, so familiar to me. Skulls gleaming white, the end of innocence, the girls dressed as boys. Phoebe was lucky last time, she wasn't narrator when Ms James watched, but today she stumbles her way through her lines, a prompt needed every minute or two. Miss Mehmet loses it, says, that's it, Phoebe, you're out, Milly's taking over as narrator. The look on her face, and while the score's not even – she's way ahead after the photo last night – I'm hot on her tail.

The punishment for stealing her part comes quickly. She posts my photo on the Year Eleven forum, a few alterations here and there, hair on my breasts and thighs. Frankenstein's bride. She changes the password for the forum to 'freak', a tactic employed to keep snooping teachers at bay. She sends an email out alerting us to the change. These highly selective schools, a breed of smart yet sneaky teens. Tricks and trolls.

A comment from LadyLucie2000 suggests, let's set up a Facebook page called Milly the Freak. Phoebe added underneath: 'Good idea!!!! I snapchatted it to Tommy at Bentleys, he's going to pass it on to all the boys' schools out of London.'

At lunch I feel the stares as I walk past the tables to the servery. The majority look down as I walk back towards them with my tray, Clondine included, but not Phoebe or Izzy. Phones out, vicious smiles on their lips. It won't be long until I'm allowed to have my own Facebook page. Once the trial's over, June said. A lot of normal things to catch up with. In it to win it. I take a seat at a table as far away from them as I can and when they leave the dining room a girl called Harriet approaches me. Asks if I'm okay, says, not all of us are like Phoebe, just try and ignore her, she'll leave you alone eventually. Sympathy. An important tool in my armour. A camouflage of my own.

It hurts, don't get me wrong, I'm not made of steel, but the heading on my photo – **Milly the FREAK, she can run but she can't hide** – makes me feel better. Phoebe still doesn't get it.

My intention of running is nil.

Hiding.
Yes.
Running.
No.

'I want you to imagine you're up on the stand, you're safe, the screen hides you from harm. The people who can see you, the jury, the lawyers and the judge, are not there to hurt you, only to listen. Identify an object to focus on in the courtroom, something that brings you comfort. I want you to look at it if any of the questions become too upsetting.'

'What if I don't know how to answer?'

'Tell the lawyers you don't understand, they'll rephrase, ask it in another way until you do.'

Mike ends the session by giving me instructions for the morning, tells me to stay in my room until Phoebe leaves for school. He told her yesterday about my minor 'procedure', that I'd be off for the rest of the week. I thank him, and I mean it.

The air in my room feels stuffier than usual, the heating in the house up high. Hard to breathe. A headache lies heavy in the centre of my forehead, makes it hard to see. I focus on laying out the clothes I'm wearing tomorrow. It isn't until they're hung over the back of the chair that I realize what I've chosen. Clothes to impress you. Trousers, not a skirt, a plain white shirt I'll tuck in like a boy. You won't be able to see me but I know you'd approve. I shouldn't be doing that. Still trying to please you.

I can't do tomorrow if I see you tonight, if you come into my room, so I sit up with the lights on, read *Peter Pan* as the hours crawl by. It's my favourite book, has been since

I was a little girl. The idea of night lights as the eyes of mothers guarding their children. I used to pray for a night light, I believed in a god back then but instead I got you.

One weekend at the refuge I watched the movie with the children. When Peter says to Wendy: 'Come with me where you'll never, never have to worry about grown-up things again,' I remember thinking, I'd like to go there.

Please.

27

I stay awake all night and when morning comes I open the cabinet door in the bathroom and wipe off the number. One becomes time. It's time.

When I'm dressed I stand in front of the full-length mirror, eyes closed. I open them only to look at my outfit, I don't look as far up as my face. On the outside I look well put together, my shirt and trousers ironed by Sevita, my shoes black, flat, a ballerina-style pump. But on the inside. A jumble sale of organs. Upside down, back to front, too much heart in my chest. Not enough.

I take the crystal Saskia gave me out of its pouch, hold it in my hand. The opposing sensations of its edges, rough and smooth, soothe me. I'm not sure I believe in it, but I put it in the pocket of my trousers anyway.

And wait.

Mike comes twenty or so minutes later, knocks on my door, tells me we're ready, Phoebe's gone.

'You should eat something,' he says.

'I can't.'

'You need to, it's going to be a long morning, even just a piece of fruit or a cereal bar.'

'Afterwards, maybe.'

'I'll grab a few things from the cupboard, you can have them in the car if you change your mind.'

Saskia's waiting in the entrance hall and as I approach her she begins to play with the zip on her coat, back and forth. Up and down. A frantic, manic noise. She stops when I stare, attempts a smile. Mike comes out of the kitchen with a plastic bag containing food I won't be able to eat. We take his Range Rover, tinted windows, I bet when he bought it, had it modified, he never thought they'd be useful in the way they are today. Shielding me from eyes that might pry, might know I'm coming.

The journey to you is hell, a private one. Nobody talks, everybody stares straight ahead, traffic lights and buses, a rubbish truck in the way. The universe saying, don't go, stay away. Mike puts on a CD, the radio too risky. A surgery overnight, performed on me. A Chinese fortune fish, red and flippy, placed in the pit of my stomach. Moves to the beat of the music, makes me feel sick for the entire fifty minutes it takes to get there. I don't want to hear Mike's words, when he says, 'We're here.'

Saskia looks round, offers me a mint. I turn away, stare out through the tint. We drive in as per June's instructions. I close my eyes as we pass the front of the building, open them again when we're deep underground. I know what the crowd looks like, I've seen it on the news. Mike never thought to remove my laptop or phone. The women you took from, in hiding, now stand in the daylight united in hatred. They trusted you. A banner held up in the crowd, an eye for an eye. Press and photographers too, not allowed inside, one official reporter only appointed by the court, a privilege. Or burden.

June waits for us by the lift in the car park, reassures me I won't see you, you're being kept in the cells on the other side of the building. The purple scar on my arm throbs as we go up in the lift, a secret hello, your way of telling me you're near. We go into a room, looks newly painted.

Cream. What will they do with our house, Mummy, a lick of paint won't be enough. Saskia asks where the bathroom is, Mike and I sit down. Four chairs in the room, soft material, a dark shade of green. I perch on the edge of mine, I don't want to feel anything against me. Behind me. Some kind of surge inside me, moving through me as if on entering the building the voltage has been turned up. Mine.

June offers me a drink of water, suggests I go to the loo while I can, but I'm not sure I trust my legs to carry me. Breathe, just breathe. A lady I've never seen before puts her head round the door.

'Five minutes, we're just waiting for the judge.'

I wipe my palms on my trousers, feel the hard lump of Saskia's crystal against my thigh. I wish I was alone, I could count my scars. Mike tells me I'll be fine, everything will be okay. I wish I believed him but the fortune fish in my stomach flips over again, predicts otherwise. I try in my mind to go to my safe place inside the hollow of the tree but when I get there, it's gone. Chopped down, taken as evidence. Saskia arrives back, the woman from earlier too.

'June, the judge is ready.'

'Grand. Okay, Milly, it's time.'

Mike stands up, I do too even though I'm not ready. You'd think I would be, I've counted the days, but something, you maybe, must have come into the room, tied sandbags round my ankles. DID YOU THINK I WAS GOING TO MAKE IT EASY FOR YOU, ANNIE? I'm not listening to you, I can't. All I have to do is answer the questions. Answer them. I follow June to the door. Both Saskia and Mike squeeze my upper arms as I pass them, one on either side. I stop, take the crystal from my pocket, show them. Saskia turns away, tearful. Mike speaks.

'We'll be here when it's over, Milly.'

The walk from the family room to the courtroom is short. My right nostril whistles, a bleed on its way. I should ask for tissues, there's time, but I can't find my voice. Saving it for court. We stop outside a large wooden door.

'They'll open it when they're ready,' June says.

I place the crystal in my pocket, she tries to engage me in small talk.

'Your birthday's in a few weeks, isn't it?'

Sweet sixteen. But I don't want to think about that so I ignore June, close my eyes, open them again when I hear movement from the door. A court usher comes out, nods at us.

'You'll be grand, Milly, take a big breath. Ready? Let's go,' June says.

The murmuring in court does nothing to disguise our footsteps. Obvious. Exposing. June leads me to a seat turned to the right of a large white screen. The chair faces the judge and jury, no executioner that I can see. Once I'm seated June walks away, sits close to the door we entered through. The whistling in my nose stops, my heartbeat kicks in. Whips up a frenzy, a juddering mess inside my chest. I see the judge, he wears a cream-coloured wig, is sat to my right on a podium, engrossed in conversation with a man in a gown, possibly one of the defence lawyers. The man whispers, the judge listens and nods. Directly in front of me sits the jury, I count seven men and five women. Twelve pairs of eyes on me, the murmuring less now. It's okay to look, Skinny told me, but don't smile, you might be accused of trying to influence them. Influence them? I'm only here to answer the lawyers' questions, nothing else.

Each jury member has a pad of paper and pen on the wooden shelves in front of them. One of them, the woman in the middle of the back row, scribbles something down, perhaps she's writing a book about me too, or playing hangman. Whose head on the rope?

I look to the left, see the prosecuting lawyers, bodies turned into each other, conversing. To the left of them, the next bench table along, sits another man in a gown, the chair next to his empty, his eyes fixed on the man talking to the judge. I'd expected to see a stenographer, fast fingers over the keys capturing every word said, but June told me they'd phased them out a few years ago, replaced by an audio-recording system operated by the court reporter.

The only person left is you.

I know from the diagrams I was shown of the court lay-out roughly where you are, further along from the defence, far to the left. I don't close my eyes, it would look odd, but I do listen, tune in to any noise that might be from you. I listen for you breathing, I know the sound well. The cigar-ettes you smoke, menthol, a gentle rasp from your throat. But no, I can't hear you. The persistent shuffling of paper and shifting of people's feet drown you out. So close to you, I am.

The man at the podium walks away, takes a seat next to the other defence lawyer. The judge looks down at the papers in front of him, looks over at me, lifts up his hand, says in a loud masterful voice, 'Court in session.'

The shuffling and shifting ceases yet I still can't hear you. Only my breath. Shaky. Too fast.

'Will the witness please stand.'

My video statement will have been played before I came in. I wonder if I'm what they expect, if I look different in the flesh. A court usher approaches me, swears me in. I choose the affirmation instead of the oath, I don't believe in a higher power.

'I do solemnly, sincerely and truly declare and affirm that the evidence I shall give shall be the truth, the whole truth –'

Remember to breathe.

'– and nothing but the truth.'

HELLO, ANNIE.

Can't breathe.

I try to ignore the hand I feel round my throat and focus on Skinny. When he stands up, faces the jury, I know what to expect. I've been tutored and schooled in the questions they'll ask. Over in a flash, he said, the last time I saw him.

'Ladies and gentlemen of the jury, we have all seen the video evidence given by the witness. I would now like to hear from her.'

He turns to face me.

'In your own words, tell the court what it was like living at home with your mother.'

An open-ended question. The lawyers explained to me they'll use questions that require a sentence or, even better, a 'story' in response. The more details, the better, Fatty said, no holds barred. So I did as I was told and practised a story to tell to the court. This one is true.

'Living with my mother was terrifying. One minute she'd be normal, doing something like making dinner, the next she'd –'

I have to take a breath before I say it out loud. It'll be the first time you've heard me talk about you. Shame floods through my body.

'It's okay,' Skinny says. 'In your own time.'

I try again.

'One minute she'd be normal, the next she'd attack me. Hurt me, very much.'

The first answer will be the worst, Fatty told me. Once you've started, you'll be fine. I find an object, focus on it. The plaque on the wall above where the jury are sitting. Skinny asks me to describe the first time I saw you hurting a child.

I tell them I saw you beat him, the first boy you took. I don't tell the jury what you said when I called you cruel for hitting his little body. You said, it's not cruel, it's love. The wrong sort of love, I replied. You punished me afterwards.

There is no.

Lash.

Such thing.

Lash.

As the wrong sort of love.

Lash.

Spittle, yours, blood, mine, alchemized in the air.

I don't tell the jury you said it was love because my lawyers told me not to, that you'd get your wish to be sentenced on the basis of diminished responsibility. Because only a person who was mad, insane, would believe what you did to be love.

Next Skinny asks me if I wanted to help the children you hurt. I pause, focus on the plaque again, flashbacks like missiles, rampaging through my mind.

Jayden. Ben. Olivia. Stuart. Kian. Alex. Sarah. Max. Daniel.

Jayden. Ben. Olivia. Stuart. Kian. Alex. Sarah. Max. Daniel.

You didn't like using their names, gave each one a number. Couldn't wait for number ten you told me on the drive to school the morning after Daniel's death. But I never forget any of their names. Or me standing at the peephole, my hand on the doorknob, trying to get to them, to stop you. Your laughter loud. The child in there with you, crying even louder.

'Does the witness need a break?' the judge asks.

SO SOON, DEAR OH DEAR. I THOUGHT I'D TAUGHT YOU BETTER THAN THAT, ANNIE.

You did.

I answer.

'No thank you.'

'I'll repeat the question, did you want to help the children your mother hurt?'

Twelve sets of eyes staring at me. Waiting.

'Yes, very much.'

'But you couldn't, could you?' Skinny continues. 'Because not only were you a victim yourself but the room used by the accused to abuse and murder the children was locked. Isn't that correct?'

'Yes.'

'Please tell the court who held the key.'

'My mother did.'

'Objection, your honour, we have evidence to suggest the witness also had access to the room.'

'What evidence have you?' the judge replies.

One of the defence lawyers stands up, speaks.

'I ask the jury to turn to page five of the report detailing the evidence gathered from the address occupied by both my client and the witness. It lists a number of children's toys found in this so-called "locked" room. Toys that belong to the witness, a teddy bear with her name sewn into the ear and a doll from a set, the remaining dolls found in the witness's bedroom. It is our position on the matter that the witness herself placed these toys in the so-called "locked" room.'

'Your honour, might I ask what proof the defence has to support this position,' Skinny counters. 'Her mother could have placed these items there without the witness's knowledge.'

'Would the defence please respond.'

I hold my breath when the defence lawyer begins to reply. Petrified by what he might say. An assortment of trump cards hidden up the sleeve of his gown.

'I find it highly unfeasible that the prosecution expect the court to believe somebody else, other than the witness, placed these toys in the room. The prosecution are asking the court to believe that my client, thus far only portrayed as evil and uncaring, placed items of comfort for the children in this locked room, out of what, out of kindness? I highly doubt that. I offer the witness as an alternative instead. Motivated by care, she placed the toys there, proving she also had access to the room.'

I breathe out. He responded as we expected him to, as my lawyers predicted he would. I know what Skinny's going to ask me next.

And I know how to answer.

CLEVER GIRL, ANNIE. HOPE IT LASTS.

'Allow me to humour the defence if I must,' Skinny continues.

He turns to face me.

'Were you the person who placed the toys listed in the evidence report into the room? Did you indeed have access to this room?'

'I did place the toys there but only when the room was empty and unlocked, I thought it would help whoever my mother brought home next. And no, when someone was in the room I didn't have access, there was only one key. She kept it on the same bunch as her car keys, took them to work every day.'

The defence lawyer who is yet to speak writes something on a piece of paper, underlines it. The other lawyer looks at it, nods. He picks the paper up, leans to his right, my left, until he's almost out of his seat. His right, my left. You. He waits a second or two, nods while looking in your direction, slides back into his seat, the paper no longer in his hands. Whatever he wrote, he left it with you. Not feeling so good any more, I didn't want to see that, the transaction between him and you, not just before we move on to the next bit. The bit that troubles me the most.

'Did you know a boy called Daniel Carrington?' Skinny asks.

'Yes, I knew him from the refuge my mother worked at.'

I look at the jury, I don't mean to. All twelve are holding their pens, poised. Ready.

'Tell the court about the night your mother brought him home, it was a Wednesday night.'

I know, I remember.

'She brought him home when I was asleep, she normally did that, brought them back at night so nobody would see. Sometimes she drugged them, so they'd be quiet.'

'So you didn't see Daniel on this particular evening?'

'I did. She woke me up.'

'Please explain to the court what happened once she woke you up.'

'She made me go to the peephole so I could see who it was.'

'She wanted to shock you, because you knew Daniel, had met him before at the refuge?'

'Yes.'

'What happened after that?'

'She went into the room, locked the door behind her and made me watch.'

'Made you watch what?'

'While she did things to him. Bad things.'

'So to clarify, your mother woke you up to make you watch her hurt a little boy she had brought home, Daniel Carrington being the boy.'

'Yes.'

'What else happened that night?' Skinny asks.

I'M STILL HERE, ANNIE. LISTENING. EVERYBODY IS.

The jury, pens moving now. Don't look at them. Safe place instead.

'She got angry with Daniel, started to hit him.'

'That must have been very hard for you to watch. You knew Daniel, you liked him.'

'I didn't watch, I closed my eyes.'

'Then what happened?'

'She came out of the room, locked the door and went to bed.'

'So your mother left Daniel in the locked room?'

'Yes.'

'Please tell the court how you knew when a child had been brought home and placed in the room opposite yours.'

'The door would be closed. It was only closed and locked if someone was in there.'

'And presumably you went to school the next day?'

'Yes, my mother drove me as usual.'

One of the defence lawyers looks to his right, a small nod of the head in your direction. Confirmation of something. But what?

'So the next time you saw Daniel was when?'

'Thursday evening.'

'And you saw him through the peephole, did you?'

'Yes.'

'Did you at any point have physical contact with Daniel when he was in the locked room? Were you able to comfort him or hold him at any point?'

'No, the door was locked the whole time. But I would have if I hadn't gone to the police on the Friday, the day after my mother killed him.'

One of the defence lawyers stands up and says, 'Objection, your honour, it's our intention to prove our client is innocent of this charge. It clearly states on the autopsy report that the cause of Daniel Carrington's death was suffocation. He was found face down on a mattress and as part of our cross-examination of the witness tomorrow we'll be exploring another avenue.'

'Overruled, the witness is merely referring to her original statement as the court would expect her to.'

Another avenue. Meaning what? You've made your lawyers hungry, haven't you? If you were playing hangman, it would be my head on the rope.

'Why would you have had contact with Daniel if you hadn't gone to the police when you did?' Skinny asks.

'It was my job to . . .'

I pause, he told me to in our practice session. Let the jury come to you, Skinny said.

'Take your time, have a sip of water if you need to,' he prompts.

I do as I'm told. He asks me to tell the court what my job was.

'It was my job to clean up afterwards.'

'After what?'

'After she killed them.'

Nine out of the twelve jurors, all of the women and four of the men, change position in their seats. Foreheads rubbed, throats cleared. A poke in the eye delivered, a blinding one. Months of disturbed sleep face them long after the trial is over. Changed for ever, by you. All of us will be.

YOU'RE DOING WELL SO FAR, ANNIE, WORKING THE CROWD, BUT WHAT ABOUT MY LAWYERS, DO YOU KNOW HOW TO WORK THEM? WHAT ABOUT TOMORROW?

I take another sip of water, try to focus on the plaque above the jury, but it keeps moving. Blurring and unblurring. Not half as reassuring as it was before.

'In your video evidence you claimed your mother killed Daniel. How were you to know this if you didn't have access to the room?' Skinny continues.

'I saw her do it through the peephole.'

'Objection, your honour.'

'Overruled, let the witness continue.'

'You saw what exactly?' Skinny asks.

'On the Thursday evening, the day after she brought Daniel home, she went upstairs to the room.'

'The room she called the playground?'

'Yes. She didn't ask me to go with her and watch, normally she would, so after a while I went up.'

'Why did you?'

'I was worried about Daniel, I wanted to help him so I went upstairs and looked through the peephole.'

'Please tell the court what you saw.'

Can't get the words out.

The room starts to swim a little, as do the edges of the faces in front of me. Hands holding pens. Nail varnish. I want them to stop writing. What are they writing about? Me? I'm not the one they should be writing about.

'Shall I repeat the question?' Skinny asks.

'Yes please,' I reply.

'What did you see your mother doing when you looked through the peephole on the Thursday night, the night after she brought Daniel home?'

'I saw my mother holding a pillow over his face. I tried to get into the room but she'd locked it from the inside.'

I can feel tears building up, I can see him. Daniel. Asking for his mummy. Tiny he was, on the bed.

'It's clear the witness is upset, perhaps you would benefit from a break at this point?' the judge asks.

'I want it to be over.'

'I'm sure you do, but are you able to continue?' he asks, dipping his head and looking over his glasses at me.

I reply, yes, because I owe it to Daniel, and to the others.

'Please tell the court how long your mother held the pillow to Daniel's face for.'

'A long time. Long enough to kill him.'

'Objection, your honour, the witness is not a medical expert therefore cannot be permitted to make a judgement on how long it might take for an individual to die.'

'Sustained, would the jury please dismiss the witness's last comment.'

'Can you tell the court about the last time you saw Daniel on the Thursday night. Where was he and what was he doing?' Skinny asks.

'Lying on the bed, not moving. Mum had gone down to

the living room. I tried to call to him through the peephole but he didn't respond, he never moved again, that's how I knew he was dead.'

'And the very next day you went to the police and reported your mother.'

'Yes, Daniel was too much. I wanted it to stop, I wanted it all to be over.'

I hear somebody exhale to my left. You. Trying to unnerve me maybe, another piece on the chessboard moved. A bishop or king.

Skinny goes on, questions me about how you controlled me, made me afraid. The torch you held to my face while whispering threats; the sleep deprivation; the psychological torment through the games you played; the physical attacks. The night-time episodes too. Members of the jury flinch and blink as they hear the extent of it. I knew Skinny would do this, he told me it was to illustrate to the court, to show that you are indeed sane, able to sustain these methods over years, all the while holding down a respectable job. When I tell the court about where you made me put the bodies, the cellar, all twelve of the jurors this time shift. Disturbing. Disturbed.

I know I'm doing okay because we're heading towards the last few questions and I haven't tripped up yet. Your voice is silent now. I'm hanging on.

Skinny faces the jury and says, 'Let us not forget that the witness you see on the stand is a child who was groomed and sexualized from a very young age, in a household where one child, a son, had already been placed in care.'

HE WAS TAKEN.
He wanted to be.

'Objection, your honour, where is this heading?'

'Yes, I agree, could the prosecution please remain on the matter in hand.'

'Could the witness please remind the court how old she is?' Skinny asks.

'Fifteen.'

'Fifteen, ladies and gentlemen. And could you please tell the court how old you were when your mother began sexually abusing you?'

'Objection, your honour.'

'Sustained, this has no relevance to the case.'

I was five. It was the evening of my fifth birthday party.

'No further questions, your honour.'

'In that case, witness dismissed.'

June tells Mike and Saskia I was 'grand', did really well. They both look relieved and agree to have me back here tomorrow at nine. When we drive out I close my eyes again, open them a few streets later. We eat lunch when we get home, afterwards I tell them I'm going to lie down, they nod. Sleep as long as you need, we'll wake you if you haven't come down for dinner, Mike says. When I checked my phone in the car there was a message from Morgan, she'd bunked off school for the day, could she come and see me in the evening. I replied telling her she could come over earlier, that I'd call her and let her know when. I call her as soon as I get into my room, knowing Mike and Saskia are at the front of the house. I tell her to hurry. She arrives on the balcony in minutes, breathless, makes a joke about being as unfit as her nana. We lie top to tail on my bed, she wriggles non-stop, her feet in my face. I tickle them, threaten to bite off her toes if she doesn't stop. She laughs, says, like to see you try.

I wouldn't, I reply in my head, sitting up.

'How come you're off school as well?' she asks.

'I had to go to court, answer some questions about my mum.'

'Why? Thought you hadn't seen her for years.'

Another lie told. The exhaustion of trying to remember who knows what.

'They wanted to ask me what she was like when I was little.'

'What was she like?'

'I don't want to talk about it.'

'How come no one knew what she was doing?'

'She was clever. Spectacular.'

'In what way?'

'People liked her, trusted her. She knew how to fool them.'

'You remember all that from when you were little?'

'Yeah, I suppose so, and from reading about it in the news.'

'When your dad died, you must have felt pretty lonely without any brothers or sisters.'

I nod, it's true. I was lonely when Luke left. I'm glad I won't be questioned about him in court, the jury would wonder why he found a way to escape sooner and I didn't. All the fights he got into, the stealing. He did anything he could to be taken away, punished in a place kinder than home. Anything but tell the truth about you, the shame he felt, what you did to him for years.

'What was it like where you used to live?' Morgan asks.

'Why?'

'Was it really different from here?'

'It was in the country, surrounded by trees. There were birds everywhere, I'd watch them for hours.'

'What sort of birds?'

'Starlings.'

A murmuration of starlings.

'Like a swarm, they moved in perfect unison, dipping and rising as if they were one. A secret language, a tilt of a wing, a flick of a feather. They flew up, flew down, flew all around, they never stopped.'

'A secret language? Like squawking and stuff?'

'No, something more beautiful, more subtle.'

'Why were they always moving like that, up and down?'

'So the bigger birds wouldn't catch them.'

'Do you reckon that's why your mum got caught, from not moving around enough?'

'Maybe.'

'Do you ever feel bad, like, I know none of it was your fault but it's still your mum, isn't it?'

'They come to me at night.'

'Who does?'

'Ask me to help them, but I can't.'

'Who are you talking about? You're being weird, I don't like it. You're scaring me.'

I'm just being me.

'Let's talk about something else, Mil. Tell me another story, another one about the birds where you lived.'

Morgan's face soothes me, her freckles, pale, not brown, a peaceful feeling when I look at her. I move up to the top end of the bed, so we're lying next to each other.

'Ready?' I ask.

'Yep.'

'It was late at night. I was washing my hands at the sink in my bedroom. I heard something behind me, scraping at the window.'

'Were you scared?'

246

'No, I turned round and it was there.'

'What was?'

'It was staring at me, eyes wide as can be, saucers surrounded by white.'

'What was?'

'An owl, through the window. It turned its head all the way round to let me know.'

'Let you know what?'

'It had seen what I'd done.'

'What do you mean? What had you done?'

'What I was told to.'

'By who?'

'It doesn't matter.'

'Then what happened?'

'It flew away. The things it saw, the things I did, too horrible for it to stay.'

She bursts into laughter, tells me I'm full of nonsense, I should be an actress.

'I haven't finished the story yet.'

'What, now you're going to tell me it came back?'

'No, it never came back but I think of it often, the shape of its face, a love heart. It looked into my window then left, flew away.'

What it saw was too ugly to love.

28

I don't remember much about getting to the court today, the drive there. The room painted cream. I'm back on the stand, one of the defence lawyers facing me. Beelzebub. I look closer but there's nothing to see, a serious face in a gown and a suit is all, his wedding finger naked, no ring. Single? Divorced? I doubt he has a child of his own tucked up at home in a crib. How could he when he's defending you?

What he does is subtle, he's better than my lawyers thought he was, much better, a slow build. I don't even notice where he's going until he gets there.

Throat.

Mine.

'Do you like children, enjoy playing with them?'

'Yes.'

'That's how you got to know Daniel Carrington, isn't it?'

'I'm not sure I understand.'

'You played with him at your mother's workplace, didn't you?'

'Once or twice, yes.'

'Once or twice? I've statements here, one from Daniel's mother and another from the woman who lived in the room next to hers at the refuge. They both corroborate you played with Daniel multiple times over a period of weeks, that you cared greatly for him, used to bring him treats. Is that true?'

The trial's not mine, not publicly anyway, yet I hear a choir start up in my head.

There's a dead man walking.

His questions are familiar, I've practised them, but today after staying up all night hiding from you again, I can't remember how to answer.

'Would the witness please respond. Did you or did you not play with Daniel multiple times over a period of weeks? A simple yes or no will do.'

'Yes.'

I look like a liar now, the jury write in their pads. A stitch inside me comes loose, is unpicked. A small amount of stuffing slides out. A lot more when he suddenly shifts the direction of his questions. Veers off course. Tactics. Dirty.

'When your older brother was taken into care, why didn't you tell the social worker who interviewed you that he was being abused by your mother? Why did you lie?'

Skinny is up on his feet immediately, challenges the defence.

'Objection, your honour, an outrageous claim, the witness was four years old when she was interviewed.'

'Sustained. This bears no relevance to the case and is a timely reminder to the defence that you are interviewing a minor.'

For weeks and weeks we drove to see you in the secure unit, Luke, but you kicked off, refused to come out of your room, wouldn't let Mum or me near you. Braver than me. I'm sorry I didn't tell them, Luke, but neither did you. I was scared, she persuaded me she was playing nice games with you, that you enjoyed them. You were diagnosed with a conduct disorder, she tried to convince the professionals to let you come home, that it wasn't your fault, probably a delayed reaction to our dad leaving. You smashed the common room at the unit to pieces the night after we left and the professionals said, no, it was safer for everyone if you remained at the secure unit. I wish I had told them, I wish I'd known how to, because things at home got so much scarier after that. I was to be her little helper from then on but I wasn't enough for her. I wasn't a boy.

The defence lawyer looks at the judge and says, 'I'd like to ask the witness about her statement claiming she saw her mother kill Daniel Carrington.'

The judge looks over at me, asks if I'm ready. I have to say yes, the only way out is through, Mike's words ringing in my head.

'Yes, I'm ready,' I reply to the judge. He nods and tells the defence to continue.

'You said you saw your mother kill Daniel.'

'Yes, I did, I think so. He didn't move after she left the room.'

'You "think" so. You said in your video evidence you saw your mother kill all nine children. Are you now saying you can't be sure whether or not she did kill Daniel?'

'I am sure, it's just hard to explain.'

IT IS, ISN'T IT, ANNIE.

You've been quiet so far, while Luke was being mentioned, but not now. Leaning forward in your seat, waiting.

'What's hard to explain?' the defence lawyer asks.

Another stitch unpicks, more stuffing leaks out. My mouth. Dry. I reach for the glass of water on the table to my right, spilling it, my hands shaking. On the edge. Me. I am.

'He wasn't moving so she must have killed him,' I reply.

'But you can't be sure, can you? Daniel's death was recorded as suffocation, could this not have been accidental after being left on the mattress with injuries rendering him immobile? Therefore, not directly at the hands of my client.'

'No, I don't think so. I'm not sure.'

'There seems to be a lot you aren't sure about today. I wonder what you would say if I asked you about the spare key to the room where the children were kept, the key my client claims you had access to.'

'Objection, your honour, again, the witness is not on trial here,' Fatty counters.

'Sustained, could the defence focus on questioning the witness rather than wondering out loud or providing the court with a commentary.'

The lawyer nods, walks towards me.

'When you last saw Daniel, where was he?'

'On the bed in the room she called the playground.'

'Can you describe what position he was lying in, please.'

'On his back, I mean on his front, he was on his front. Lying face down on the mattress.'

The jury's eyes pierce through me. Scribble, scribble. Liar, liar, they're thinking. Pants on.

'Which one was it? On his front or on his back?'

I'm holding the crystal Saskia gave me, my knuckles crack as I clench my fist round it. All I can think is that June was right to play devil's advocate: what if she can't cope. What if the reality of being on the stand is too much for her.

The judge speaks again, asks as he did yesterday, does the witness need a break?

If it's lucky, yes please.

'No thank you.'

The lawyer continues.

'So just to clarify, what position was Daniel lying in?'

There are eight little somethings hidden in the cellar and if the ninth little something also dies. Whose fault is it?

'On his front, face down,' I reply.

'And you're sure this time?'

I nod.

'Please can the witness answer the question out loud.'

'Yes, I'm sure.'

In the same way my silence unnerves Phoebe, yours unnerves me. Confident. That's how you feel. You expect me to mess up but secretly you'd like me not to, I expect. A testament to how well you taught me, able to hold my own while expert lawyers try to unravel me. Loosen my finger-tips on the edge of a building. A long way to fall.

'My client claims that the day after she brought Daniel home, a Thursday, she went to work and stayed there late unexpectedly.' He turns to me. 'You got the school bus home, the driver confirmed this, he remembered because as you said yesterday your mother usually drove you, meaning you were home alone for over two hours before your mother returned to the house. Is that correct?'

The nod of his head yesterday, in your direction, when I said you usually drove me. Heat being turned up. Can't breathe. Very well. You. Me. Both witnesses, we were there. I saw you. My chest feels tight. Head, busy. I ask him to repeat the question.

A lady in the second row of the jury circles something

in her notepad, looks up, her eyes locked on me. I look away, try to focus on what he might ask next but there's no point, these aren't questions we prepared for. I never told my lawyers I was alone in the house, they never asked, it's not me who's on trial, there was no need to check whether she drove me home that day or if I took the bus. The faces of my lawyers are stony, not at all at ease. I'm not doing so well today, and I'm sorry to say, things could get worse, a lot worse, if I tell the truth. Release the carrier pigeon trapped in my chest, let it do its job. Deliver its message.

The defence lawyer asks me again if I was home alone with Daniel on the Thursday afternoon when he was still alive and in the room.

'Yes,' I reply.

Skinny and Fatty exchange glances, I know what they're thinking, they're thinking this is news to us, really bad fucking news and now is not a good time to be finding out new information. The defence lawyer smells it from me, the urge, the need to disclose. He's seen it before, massage the back while he continues to go for the throat. He lowers and softens his voice, reassures me, tries to reel me in.

'Did you try to open the door to the room Daniel was in?'

I'm about to say yes, yes, I did, but somebody coughs. You. I know it was you, I know how your everything sounds. But why did you? Are you worried about what my answer might be, worried that the game will be over in minutes if I can't hold on any longer, if I crumble under the pressure. You'd be so disappointed. An anticlimax. And a reflection on you, my teacher. Don't worry, I won't, though I'd be lying if I said I hadn't thought about it. The temptation of telling the truth, how that might taste. How that might feel. And whether it would be worth it, or whether I'll still have to live with a snake and the ghosts of nine little somethings playing at my feet. Regardless.

'The witness looks distracted, I'll repeat the question. Did you try to open the door?'

'Yes, I tried, but it was locked.'

'So at no point did you enter the room where Daniel was?'

'No.'

'You never went into the room, you never touched Daniel, tried to comfort him?'

'I did, yes.'

'You did which? You entered the room or you tried to comfort him?'

'I tried to comfort him.'

'In what way?'

HELLO, ANNIE.

The crystal drops from my hand, lands under the table where the glass of water sits, the sound reverberates off the wood of the stand. Too many eyes to count now, all focused on me. I look over at June, she signals for me to leave it but I want to bend down, pick it up, so I can hide, never come up.

'In what way did you comfort Daniel?'

A pit bull, the lawyer is. Teeth latched on to flesh. On to anything it can.

'I spoke to him through the peephole.'

'He was alive at this point then, when you were talking to him through the peephole?'

'Yes.'

'What did you say to him?'

'That I was sorry and it would soon be over, that every-thing would be okay.'

True.

'What would soon be over? How could you know that, you're not your mother, are you? You had no idea how long he would be kept there for.'

'I wanted to make him feel better.'

True.

'What was Daniel doing at this time?'

'Crying, asking for his mummy.'

True.

'And at no point while Daniel was in the house did you touch him?'

'No.'

'If I told you the forensic expert we consulted found evidence of your DNA on Daniel's clothing, what would you say to that?'

'Objection, your honour, the witness had prior contact with the victim at the refuge. DNA could easily have transferred on to the clothing then.'

'Agreed, sustained.'

Without whistling or warmth, my nose begins to bleed. A red droplet rolls down over my lips, my chin, lands on the wood of the podium. Everybody's staring, look, there she is, the daughter of a murderer covered in blood. Take her away, take her down, is what they could say. I hear Fatty asking for a recess.

'Does the witness require one?' the judge asks.

I cover my nose, an usher gives me a box of tissues, I feel light-headed. Can't remember what I was saying. The truth. No. Yes. I want to tell the truth.

'Your honour, can't the court see the witness's distress?' Fatty stands up and says.

'Yes, but I'm also mindful these questions must be asked and the sooner we do that the sooner the witness can be dismissed and go home,' the judge replies.

I want to go home now.

YOU DON'T HAVE A HOME ANY MORE, YOU MADE SURE OF THAT, ANNIE.

I hold a wad of tissues against my nose, take a deep breath and wait for the next question.

'So Daniel's in the room crying, asking for his mummy. Then what happened?'

'I heard my mother's car pull into the drive so I went downstairs.'

'Did you and your mother speak at all?'

'No. When she came into the house she walked past me, went up the stairs and into the room where Daniel was.'

'Did she unlock the door first or was it already unlocked?'

'It was. It was locked, that's what I mean, she opened it. She had the keys in her hand as she passed me.'

'And then what did you do?'

'After a while I went upstairs.'

'And through the peephole you claim you saw my client holding a pillow over Daniel's face, is that correct?'

'Yes, he didn't move afterwards.'

'How long did you stay at the peephole for?'

'I'm not sure.'

'Roughly. Minutes? Hours? The whole night?'

'No, only a few minutes maybe. When she came out of the room we went down for dinner.'

True.

'And you went back later on, did you? To the peephole.'

'Yes, I went to comfort him.'

True.

'But he was dead, you said you saw your mother kill him. Why would you go back if he was already dead?'

'I don't know.'

'You weren't sure if he was dead, that's what you're saying, isn't it?'

'No. He was dead, he wasn't moving.'

I see the second defence lawyer being passed a piece of paper from my left. From you. My insides untether, a hot-air balloon straining at its moorings. He reads it then asks the judge if he can pass it to his colleague. If relevant to the questions being asked, then yes, the judge replies. The lawyer in front of me walks away, collects the piece of paper, reads it, nods. I look out at the jury, Daniel's ghost is standing next to them. He's shaking his head, hangs it down and begins to cry. Two peas in a pod we are, you said one night, Mummy. So alike. Sticks and stones may break my bones but names can never hurt me.

False.

The lawyer walks back over to me, the piece of paper slid along the bench from you now in his hands, then says, 'The forensic expert concluded that Daniel's death could have occurred during the time period you were alone in the house with him, not necessarily after my client returned home as was previously thought. What would you say to that?'

'Objection, your honour.'

'Overruled, let the witness answer.'

The bleed in my nose has stopped but a red polka dot of blood must have landed before I was given the tissues. A stain on the front of my shirt like ink on chromatography paper. One of the women in the jury looks close to tears. She's a mother, I bet. I'm sorry, I am.

'I don't know. I'm not sure.'

The lawyer pauses, looks down at the note in his hands. Looks up at me, makes me wait. Ready when he's ready, torture is best served slow. He walks closer towards me, brown shoes like Prof West's, a navy pinstripe suit visible under his gown. He nods as he walks, stops directly in front of me, then says, 'I can see why you might not be sure. It's a tricky one, isn't it? There's the matter of the spare key your mother claims you had access to, your DNA being found on Daniel's clothing, and now the time of his death potentially being when you were alone in the house. I think, given the facts I've just laid out, I'm entitled to, perhaps even obliged, to ask you –'

Skinny interrupts with, 'Objection, your honour, the defence are being inflammatory.'

'Overruled. But I urge the defence to tread carefully.'

The lawyer nods, but something about the way he's standing, legs wide apart, shoulders pulled back, indicates that the last thing he's thinking about doing is treading carefully. It's glory he's after. It's me he's after. His eyes narrow as they look at me, he breathes in, his chest full. His Ulysses moment. Then he asks it, the question he's been building up to all along.

'It wasn't my client who killed Daniel, was it? Tell the court what really happened the night of his death, tell the truth.'

Nobody hears my answer, drowned out by an eruption of 'objections' from both Skinny and Fatty. Shouts of 'objection, your honour, this is intimidation of a witness'. Both on their feet, both saying, she's a minor, she's not on trial. The jury look confused, pens no longer poised but being chewed, a man in the front row holding his hands up in a 'who knows' gesture. June is also on her feet, not looking half as 'grand' as usual. It's only you I can't see. Smiling though, I bet, enjoying the chaos you've managed to cause, to orchestrate.

I lied.

That's what my answer was.

I say it again.

'I lied.'

It takes a further two times, I lied, I lied, for the judge to hold up his hand, silence the court. 'Let the witness speak,' he says.

This is it, Mummy, the moment you were waiting for, where I crack. Where you win.

'I lied.'

Nobody but the defence lawyer moves a muscle. No shifting of feet, no crossing and uncrossing of legs, no scribbling of notes. The lawyer walks over to me again, rests his hand on the wood in front of me, a friendly gesture, but he's no friend, he's hungry. Wants feeding. Alphabet spaghetti served in the shape of lies he's slowly squeezing out of me, the key witness. I can see that night so clearly, I was there. I know what happened.

'What did you lie about?' he asks.

I nod, I can tell them, it's okay. I tried to help Daniel, I did the best I could. I wanted him to be safe dilly dilly, out of harm's way. True. I tell them I'm sorry. So sorry. True. The jurors' faces, frozen. June. My lawyers. The judge.

'What did you lie about?' he asks again.

'I lied to Daniel when I told him through the peephole

everything would be okay, I knew it wouldn't but I told him that anyway. I let him down. That's how I lied.'

I begin to cry, salty tears stained red as my nose begins to run. I can see the defence lawyer's disappointment, his face crumples a little. It's not dinner time yet, you know.

Now fuck off.

He removes his hand, continues to look at me. He can look all he likes but he can't prove a thing and his time is up, he'll be done for harassing a minor if he keeps going and he knows it. He walks away, sits back down and says the words I've been waiting to hear.

'No further questions, your honour.'

'In that case, the witness is free to leave the stand.'

A wave. Raw. Sadness washes over me as I'm dismissed. I don't move, I look at the screen. I want to run to you, crawl up inside you back into your womb. Rewrite a history where this time you'd love me normally. Shiny and new. The judge speaks again, June beckons for me to come.

'You're free to go, Milly,' he says.

He's tired too. His wig, horse-hair, heavy. Hot. He says my name, my new name, out loud.

Against the rules. She's on it, like a hound on a fox.

'Her name is Annie.'

All heads pivot towards you. You don't sound deranged, like the monster they expect. You sound like a mother, one who cares. It takes all my resolve, something more, not to run to you. The courtroom struggles to process the judge's mistake, murmurs become voices, grow in sound.

'Silence in court,' he says.

It takes longer than before for the room to quieten, his power, his credibility less. Not yours though, four words from you is all it takes. Your voice, a nimbus cloud hanging low in the air, threatening hail. A storm.

June takes my arm, I stop to pick up the crystal then she leads me out of the courtroom. I don't hear a choir any more, no song in my head, your voice instead saying my name. ANNIE.

I'm back in the room painted cream, you follow me there too. Mike and Saskia see my face, and my shirt.

'Just a nosebleed,' I say. 'I'm going to the bathroom to clean up.'

'Shall I come with you?' Saskia offers.

'No, it's okay, thank you.'

'We'll wait for you here,' Mike adds.

I nod.

The door of the toilet seals with a lock, slides to the right. I reach into my pocket, the Black Tourmaline. Can't on my ribs, shirt, white. Trousers down. Thigh instead. I have to press hard, the rough edge, not the smooth, scrape it across the skin. I carve out an A. Like coming up on a drug, a whip. The pain takes me there, it takes me to you.

A IS FOR ANNIE.

Yes, I'll always be Annie to you but to others I'm Milly. Siamese twins inside me, at war.

Good me.

Bad me.

Proud of me, are you? I played the game, I might even have won, Mummy.

When I get back to the family room June says she'll be following up with the court about how I was treated by the defence. Mike calls them bastards, job or no job, he says. It's okay, I tell him, it's over now. Saskia looks relieved. June sees us out to the car park and says things are likely to move quickly, the verdict could be as early as next week.

Sit tight.

Later on at home I go to Mike's study, he wants to see me before the weekend kicks off, check I'm okay after court. Phoebe's there when I arrive, she's still grounded for breaking curfew, the punishment for the party pushed back until after the hockey tour. She's bargaining with Mike, trying to persuade him to let her go out.

'Come on, it's Friday,' she says, 'everyone's going to the cinema.'

'No,' he replies, 'you're grounded until Monday.'

'You're being so stupid, Dad.'

'I think it was you that did the stupid thing.'

'And you've never made a mistake?'

'I'm not getting into this again, Phoebe, Monday it is and that's the last I want to hear about it. Now if you don't mind, darling, I need to catch up with Milly about something.'

'Yeah, great. Nice one, Dad. Thanks a lot.'

Another killer stare as she passes.

He closes the door, says, I'm afraid I'm not very popular right now, then smiles, asks me to take a seat.

'I won't keep you long, it's been a long day already and you look exhausted. How are you feeling now it's over?'

'I'm not sure, it doesn't feel real yet.'

'That's understandable. I wanted to say how proud I am of you and how sorry I am the defence treated you that way. I feel partly responsible to be honest.'

'Why? It wasn't your fault.'

'No, but perhaps we could have prepared you better

than we did. Perhaps we should have been a bit more up front with you.'

'Up front about what?'

'June called me one weekend to let me know your mother had been saying a few things about the night Daniel was killed.'

The conversation I overheard when I was in the alcove.

'We didn't think we should tell you, the lawyers weren't supposed to broach it in the way they did.'

'What sort of things was she saying?'

'Utter nonsense, the judge quashed her claims immediately. I just wish you hadn't had to go through what you did today.'

'I'm all right, honestly. You've helped me a lot, Mike.'

'I hope so, and at least now we can focus on you, on the work that needs to be done to help you heal.'

'Will you do it with me?'

'As much of it as I can, yes.'

'As much of it as you can?'

'Don't worry about that today, Milly. All you need to worry about is getting a good night's sleep, you deserve it.'

Do I?

I fall asleep fast, two nights without does that, it forces your eyes closed, takes you to places you don't want to go. A little boy at the end of my bed, eyes wide and frightened. I can't breathe, he says, I can't breathe.

Up eight. Up another four.
The door on the right.

I swear to tell the truth, the whole truth.
And nothing but the truth.
This, along with the birthday plans you had for me,
is the other reason I left when I did.
You were at work, I was alone in the house, not through
the peephole but inside the room.
A spare key, I knew where you hid it.
His tiny body curled up on the bed, in the corner.
He stirred as I came in, I closed the door behind me.
Skin pale, a lack of fresh air. Black circles under his eyes,
he asked for his mummy. Yes. You'll see her soon, I told him.
His brown eyes, wet with relief.
I held him close to my body, warmed his blood through.
Your voice in my head, the things you said to his mummy so she
would give him to you.
What if your husband comes after you, Susie? What if he
hurts your son? Worse even. I have a contact in
America who works in adoption.
A loving family awaits, a better life for Daniel.
Tell no one.
I gave him a teddy to hold, one of mine, name sewn in the ear.
Close your eyes, I told him, make a wish. I held him tight
through the worst, as the air left his lungs.
As I suffocated him.
You were outside the room when I opened the door, back earlier than
expected, your turn to watch through the peephole.

You looked at me in a way I hadn't seen before.
That's my girl, you said. Proud.
I never told you, Mummy, that I did it to save him.
Not to please you.
When I said I told the police everything, almost everything.
I meant it.

29

It was the way she said it yesterday, when we'd finished Sunday brunch with Mike and Saskia and we were going up to our bedrooms. So how was your little procedure anyway, she asked, what actually was it? It was fine thanks but I'd rather not talk about it. She smiled, nodded, said, must be difficult for you, not being able to talk about things, *lots* of things. The emphasis on 'lots'. An uneasy feeling, a seed planted in my stomach. Pandora's Box being nudged open. She knows. What does she know? How can she? Mike and me have been so careful, haven't we?

Today is the last day to enter our portfolios for the art prize, the winner is to be announced next week. The first thing I do when I get to school this morning is send MK an email. We arrange to meet at the end of the day and when I arrive she tells me I'm a little behind.

'The other entrants finished last week, while you were . . . away.'

I don't want to be paranoid but it was the pause, the gap she left before finishing her sentence, as if she harbours doubt as to where I was, what I was doing. Imagining it, I must be, just as I am with Phoebe. Surely.

'Why don't you lay out all of your sketches in the order you did them and we'll whittle them down to the five you need.'

As I lay out the sketches of you I think of the trial still going on, you sat in a chair, handcuffed, facing life in prison, no contact with me. You don't cope well with loss. Losing Luke changed everything, your desires turned darker, more fatal. You got bored of it just being me and you, took Jayden, the first boy, less than a year after Luke left. Love is a lubricant and, though it was warped, you got it from us. Who will you get it from now? You might make the woman in the cell next to yours swallow her tongue. There's always possibilities you said, opportunities for mischief.

MK's voice interrupts my thoughts.

'Wow, when they're laid out like that you can really see.'

'Really see what?' I ask her.

'The journey, as if each one's a piece in a puzzle.'

Then she asks me something strange.

'Are you feeling more secure now you're staying with the Newmonts?'

The sketches are heavily disguised, face smudged, eyes a different colour from yours. It's not possible to recognize the subject, I'm certain.

'I'm not sure what you mean.'

She shakes her head and says, 'It doesn't matter. I'd go with those two for definite, that one at the end, and you choose the other two, perhaps some that demonstrate a real depth of shading.'

Somebody says goodnight as they pass the door. MK says, hang on, Janet, is that you? But the corridor door opens and closes again, she can't have heard.

'Give me a second,' she says. 'I need to catch her about something.'

The room feels empty, less appealing, when she leaves. I choose the last two sketches, find myself walking over to her desk, her diary, open. A Post-it note – *order more clay*.

Her writing's glorious, all loop di loops. Loving. The *y* in the word clay is drawn long, wraps round the other letters, an inky hug. A thick piece of card is sticking out of the back page of the diary. Cream. Gold calligraphy on the front. I slide it out. A wedding invitation, names I don't know, but it's not the names that interest me it's something else, the envelope behind the invite. I turn it over, an address, an address for MK. I know where her road is, I've walked along it with Morgan. I replace both the card and the envelope, hear the door at the end of the corridor open and walk back to my sketches.

'Sorry about that. Have you made a decision?'

'Yes, these five.'

'Great choice, they'll be hard to beat, that's for sure. Janet just reminded me that the Muse gallery on Portobello Road has a fantastic exhibition of charcoal sketches on at the moment. It's a shame it's the last night, I think you'd have enjoyed it.'

'We could still go, couldn't we? Tonight? I'd have to ask Mike but he won't mind if it's for school.'

'Actually, I meant for you, you should go. I didn't mean we'd go together.'

'Oh, okay, sorry, it just sounds really great but I don't think Mike will let me go on my own.'

Anxious, a bit overprotective since court, wants me home every night until the verdict's announced.

'I'd really like to go, Miss Kemp, especially after the procedure I had last week.'

'Yes, how was that by the way?'

'It was okay, it's over now.'

'Something to be glad about, I'm sure. I'm not promising anything, I have plans tonight, but I might try and pop into the gallery around sevenish. I wouldn't mind a quick look myself. Why don't you go with Mike and if I see you there, great.'

'Okay, sure, I'll ask him. You'll be there at seven?'

'I'll try.'

Mike offers to accompany me to the gallery, I say no, it's only a short walk away. I left out the part about meeting MK, told him all of the entrants for the art prize were going. He was unsure at first but I persuaded him, I'm good at that. After everything that's been going on, I say. He nods. Understands.

Before I leave he checks I have my phone, tells me I look lovely, grown up even. I hope I haven't got it wrong, chosen the wrong dress. I wait for her outside the gallery, it'll be nice to walk in together I think. A few people drift in and out, I was a little early, so when it gets to ten past seven I've been standing there for almost twenty minutes, can barely feel my feet, pull my school coat tight round my body. I check my phone which is pointless as she doesn't have my number nor do I have hers.

When it gets to twenty past I try to stay calm, reassure myself she's just a bit late, that her artistic chaos will wrap round me when she arrives, making everything feel better. Timekeeping and discipline are the keys to success you used to say but I don't want to think about you.

'MK's nothing like you.'

'Sorry?' comes a reply.

I realize I've spoken out loud as a trio of women exit the gallery and pass by. I mumble an apology, say something about practising my lines. They smile as they remember their schooldays long gone, happy days, judging by their smiles. Or the fact that time dilutes the bad memories as I hope it will mine.

I look at my phone, twenty-five to eight. She's not coming, I know that now. When I get home I go straight to my room, hug a pillow to my chest. I long for the one from Mike's office, blue, so soft.

You whisper in my ear, remind me that you're my mummy, and what MK did was wrong. I put the duvet over my head, but your words get to me anyway and after a while I begin to listen to what you're saying, begin to agree. You're right, I know you are, what MK did wasn't nice.

I hear it when you reply, the excitement in your voice.

THAT'S MY GIRL, ANNIE. WHAT WILL YOU DO?

TELL ME, WHAT WILL YOU DO?

30

The verdict comes in on Wednesday, just under a week after I was in court. I check my phone as usual on the way back from school, three missed calls from Mike in the past half hour. I log on to the BBC news web page, your picture. The word: sentenced.

Guilty.

Guilty.

Guilty times twelve.

You go down for all nine murders, the judge passed sentence immediately. Life, no chance of parole. Mike's waiting for me by the front door, opens it as I arrive. I nod to let him know I've seen the news. He says, come here, shh, it's okay.

I thought I'd be happy, relieved. That after the trial was over I'd be able to leave behind what I did to Daniel. I did what I did to be good, to save him, yet it still makes me bad. It makes me the same as you.

Saskia comes into the hallway, rubs the spot in between my shoulder blades.

'I'm sorry, Milly. But at least it's over now, we can start planning your birthday,' she says.

When I look up I see Mike signal no with his eyes. Too soon, he means. She clocks it, looks disappointed for getting it wrong. Again.

'Whenever you feel ready then, Milly,' she says, walking away.

Mike asks me if I'd like to catch up, he's keen, the next

chapter of his book to be written I bet. The day of the verdict. I tell him no, I'd like to be alone.

I sit on the floor, my back against the end of the bed. I sit and think of you. Of the times we had. The times you sat there in your chair, no such thing as underwear. A programme on killers, brethren you said, though I'm better than them, I won't get caught. How will they catch me? You berated their inadequacies, their failings. It's because they're men, you said, being a woman gives me a shield and you do too, Mummy's little helper.

The press, the name they gave you, you'll have heard, and seen your face on the front of the newspapers. Your nickname, my favourite book, written in bold:

THE PETER PAN KILLER

You'll like it I think, the sentiment is right. Out of your hands anyway, now under lock and key. The extra details I provided to the police must have leaked to the press. The words you whispered to each limp body that lay in the room, tucked up asleep. For ever. That's what you get for leaving your mummy, your voice, through clenched teeth as you hissed in their ears though they couldn't hear any more. I tried to say to you it wasn't their choice, their mummies gave them away. No, no, no, you shouted at me, I didn't give my son away, he was taken. They're not Luke, I said, you can't replace him. You beat me black, you beat me blue for mentioning his name.

You beat me.

More disturbing than hurt is love when it's wrong. In your arms you swayed them, placed them down as if they could be broken, even more, or again. Six boys. Daniel was

274

seven but he wasn't yours. Six little princes of sorts, wrapped up in blankets, new pyjamas each time. Two little girls. You didn't care for the girls. Don't disturb me until I've finished, you used to say. Finished what?

Saying goodbye.

Every single time, that's what it was about. The rituals, the dressing of the boys in pyjamas. Pyjamas is what Luke was wearing the evening he was taken away after they discovered it was him that snuck out one night and set fire to the post office in our village, the flat above thankfully empty at the time. He was eleven years old.

Hellos are important, it's how we begin, but to steal a goodbye, not giving you the chance to hold Luke one last time before he was taken. To you that was the ultimate sin.

I'm interrupted by my bedroom door opening and Phoebe walking in. She doesn't say anything, stands there, looks down at me and stares.

'What are you looking at?' I ask.

She doesn't answer. Tiny piranhas tear at my insides.

And all the king's horses, and all the king's men.

She stares for a bit longer, then backs slowly out of the room, not bothering to close the door behind her.

I meet with Mike after dinner, he asks me how I feel about the verdict. Sick, I tell him, not how I expected to. He spoke to June, wanted to know the details of what happened in court, asks me why I never told anybody I was home alone with Daniel. I was scared, I reply, I knew my mum might try and blame me. And what about you, do you still blame yourself, he asks. Yes, I tell him, I always will. Why, he persists. Why wouldn't I, I reply. He looks at me strangely, a scrutiny of sorts, but lets it drop.

Later on I take out the remainder of my sketches of you, the ones I didn't enter into the art prize. I can't explain why it's comforting to look at you. But it is. What's not comforting is feeling Phoebe's eyes on me. Coming into my room, staring at me.

It hurts me to do it but I rip up your sketches until you're nothing more than a pile of eyes, lips and ears. I want to move on, I want a normal home filled with normal things. Mike asked me once what I wanted from life. Acceptance. That's what my answer was. To accept where I've come from and who I am, to be able to believe and prove the curious shape you twisted my heart into could be untwisted. And it will be, Milly, he replied, just wait and see. He doesn't know how curious a shape it is though. I gather up the ripped sketches, put them in the bathroom bin. An hour or so later I remove them, tape them back together.

Morgan's text comes through after midnight, are you awake, she asks, I need to see you. I tell her to come to the balcony and when she does she looks smaller than before, shrunk a size or two. I open the door. Cold air chases its way in, the jester of winter fills up each corner, dances. Jeers. Her mouth is bloody and swollen, the skin on the left-hand side of her forehead scraped, looks like a carpet burn. I take her by the hand, bring her inside, close the door and lock it. Check it twice.

'What happened?'

She shakes her head, small stiff movements, her eyes on the floor.

'I didn't know where else to go,' she replies.

Her fingers cycle the air in front of her, tying and un-tying imaginary knots. I walk over to the bedside lamp, switch it on. Her jeans are stained and a salty sour smell emanates from her, a hint of alcohol on her breath.

'Are you hurt anywhere else?'

She wipes her sleeve across her nose and straight away it runs again, a stream of clear liquid into her mouth. Her chin begins to wobble. No tears. The shock of whatever's happened stops them. I pick up the box of tissues on the floor by my bed.

'Here.'

I raise my arm to throw them to her, she flinches, cowers a little. I lower my hand, want to say, it's me, don't be afraid, but then I remember I've hurt her before.

'You can stay here tonight.'

She shakes her head.

'Yes, I'll help you, I'll make it better.'

'What if somebody comes in?'

'They won't, everybody's asleep.'

I take a pair of pyjamas from my drawer, soft cotton ones. You'd punish me for caring for her, she's not a boy, you'd say, girls don't need gentle. No, I'd reply, she's not a boy, but she's something to me.

The lamp from the light is low but when I help take off her top I see bruises beginning to form. An imprint, the outline of a shoe on the side of her ribs. I rest her hands on my shoulders as I lean down, lift each leg out of her trousers into the pyjamas. I straighten up, her hands stay on my shoulders. We stand like that for a while, facing each other. Eventually I move away, gather her clothes into a pile, put them on the chair by the balcony door.

'Sit down on the bed, I'll get a cloth for your face.'

She winces as I clean the blood from the swelling around her mouth.

'Who did it?'

'I wish he was dead,' she replies.

'Who?'

'My uncle.'

She bursts into tears, I hold her, rock us back and forth, begin to hum. *Lavender's blue, dilly dilly . . .* Her breathing calms, her tears stop.

'I love that song,' she says.

'I know. Lie down, you need to rest.'

She does without protest, turns on her side towards me, draws her knees up to her chest. I cover her with the duvet, an extra blanket. Her eyes close. She pushes one of the pillows from under her head on to the floor.

'I only have one at home,' she says.

I sit next to her on the bed, watch her face contract, relax, as she tries to forget what happened. You shall be safe, dilly dilly, out of harm's way, Morgan. I can't help with her uncle but she's different. Out of harm's way, that's what I can do. I pick up the pillow, think how much she'd like Neverland, a place where dreams are born and time is never planned, but she moves, rubs her eyes, balled-up little fists like small children when they're tired. She opens her eyes, looks up at me, at the pillow in my hand, asks me what I'm doing.

'Nothing, just putting it back on the bed.'

'I'm safe here, aren't I, Mil?'

'Yes.'

'Good,' she replies, the smallest voice.

When I wake up in the morning she's gone. Pyjamas at the foot of the bed, a tiny pile.

31

I didn't see Phoebe at home this morning but she and Izzy are the first people I see when I walk into Thursday assembly. I sit in the row behind them, a few seats to the left. I listen to the conversations going on around me, any hint people might know, but it's the usual. Hairstyles and boys, plans for Christmas, who still needs tickets for the play. The organ starts, we stand up as the teachers file in on to the stage. A younger girl, from Year Nine I think, gives a presentation about 'paying it forward', the good things we can do over the festive period to help the less fortunate. She gets a strong round of applause. Ms James stands up to deliver the weekly announcements, talks about the proposed refurb of the senior common room, if anybody's interested in fundraising please see Mrs McDowell in the office. A couple of other items related to the running order of the performance days for our play are detailed, and the last announcement is:

'The recipient of this year's Sula Norman Art Prize is Milly Barnes in Year Eleven.'

The applause is slow, better than none. Ms James goes on to say that my name will be etched in gold paint on the awards board in the stairwell leading up to the Great Hall, and to see Miss Kemp for the rest of the details. I feel uncomfortable, not because of the public praise but because I haven't seen MK since the day she was supposed to meet me at the gallery. And because I can sense Phoebe's eyes on me. When I look over at her, she immediately looks away.

MK finds me in the library during lunch, trying to work on a history essay, but I've read the same sentence over and over again. She smiles as she approaches me.

'Congratulations, I had a feeling you'd win. Sula's parents and the gallery owner loved your sketches, it was a unanimous decision.'

'Thank you.'

'You should be very proud, especially with everything that's —'

She stops but it's too late, the look on her face, the telltale signs of her adjusting each layer of beads round her neck, her rings next.

'Everything that's what?'

She sits down next to me. I was right to suspect when I saw her on Monday.

'That's why you didn't come.'

'Come where?' she asks.

'To the gallery. You said you'd meet me at seven, I waited for over half an hour.'

'You mean Monday? Oh, Milly, I said I'd try but couldn't promise anything.'

'It's fine, I understand.'

'It's not like that, my friend came over earlier than expected, we went out. I forgot. I'm sorry.'

She breathes in through her nose, lets it out slowly, her cheeks inflate. She leans in towards me, the scent of lavender.

'I had a feeling something was up, Milly. The sketches; the emails; the present you tried to give me; you being off school. I spoke to Ms James again and she ended up telling me about, well, where you're from.'

I count the books on the shelf above her head. I get to eleven, then she says, 'I know about your mum, Milly.'

'That's why you don't want to be my guidance teacher any more.'

'That's absolutely not the reason but it might have been helpful for me to know.'

'You signed your emails MK.'

'Sorry, I don't understand.'

'I thought you cared.'

'I do care but I sign all my emails MK, have done for years. I'm sorry if you felt I was misleading you. I'd have been more careful if I'd known.'

A banner pops up, the upper-right corner on the screen of my laptop, an alert for an email: 'New post added on Year 11 forum.' I click on the link, it takes a while to open, an image downloading.

The image is a picture of you.

The title: 'Ding dong the Wicked Witch who SHOULD be dead.'

Underneath, two thumb icons. One facing up, one facing down. Vote whether you agree. Seventeen votes so far. One thumb, redundant.

I slam the lid of my laptop down, stand up, my chair tips over, crashes on to the ground. Move. Can't. Walk. Can't.

MK stands ups, says, 'Milly, what is it?'

Wicked witch. SHOULD be dead. Ding dong. You. You should be dead, that's what they're voting on and I know who'll be next.

The librarian comes over and asks if everything's okay.

'I'm not sure. Milly? Is everything okay?'

'I need to go.'

'Go where? What's happened?'

'I can't talk about it, I'm sorry,' I say, gather up my things and walk away.

'Sorry about what? Where are you going? I haven't told you about the art prize yet.'

I go straight to the sick bay, a hidden typewriter in my head punching out the words as I walk: Phoebe knows. Phoebe knows.

And soon everybody will, if they don't already.

'I don't feel very well, Miss Jones, please can I go home?'

'You certainly look a bit peaky. Any idea what it is?'

'I think it's a migraine.'

'Yes, I remember reading on your medical form you suffered from them. I'll need to call the Newmonts, they're your guardians, aren't they?'

'Yes.'

The clock on the wall has a gentle tick, a trance-like rhythm like the one in my bedroom the night the police came. I have the same feeling I had then, the waiting, the wishing it was over. Only this time I don't know what the 'it' is.

'That's fine, I spoke to Mr Newmont. Either he or his wife will be home in an hour or two, the housekeeper's there at the moment. Will you manage the walk back?'

I nod.

'Good, well feel better, get some rest and lots of fluids.'

Sevita's waiting for me when I get there.

'Hello, Miss Milly, you like some lunch?'

'No thank you, I'm going straight to bed, I don't feel very well.'

'Okay, I'm in the laundry.'

I see her hand cross her chest as she walks away from

me, a Hail Mary. A prayer for me, or her. Home alone. With me.

I pace in my room for a bit, need to think clearly. Does Phoebe know? Was the post on the forum directed at me or just a sick game in response to the trial verdict? Cornered. Me. No way out. Fight, flight. Where would I go if I ran? There's nowhere for someone like me to go.

I have to find out what Phoebe knows and if anyone else does. Who would she have told? Clondine? Izzy? All of the girls in my year maybe but I saw some of them on my way out of school and nothing happened. They'd have said something if they knew. I sit down on my bed, try to still my mind, all the while feeling sand in the timer slipping away. I stand up, pace back and forth again. Think, damn it, think. A golden nugget of memory lands when I see the top corner of my laptop poking out of my school bag.

The door I open I shouldn't, it's not mine. One of the house rules, bedrooms are private, it's forbidden to go into each other's without permission. Mike. His idea of domestic utopia but there's nobody here to ask so I give myself permission. Her room is a cliché, I've been in before over half-term. Posters and pink, a sweet smell in the air. Candy-floss. Caramel. Sugar and spice. Polaroid strips of her and her friends sit Blu-Tacked on the wall above her desk. Fairy lights the shape of hearts hang over the foot of her bed. A grotto. A sleigh for a princess, a queen made of ice. Sticky tubs of lip gloss stand tall like stones from Stonehenge on her bedside table, you never know who you'll meet in your dreams. I do.

I find what I'm looking for in the middle drawer of the desk. I'm lucky, it could've been at school with her but I know she hardly takes it, prefers her phone, that's where most of the action happens. I slide the laptop out, power it up, her email account open on the screen, one new message. I can't risk reading it – she'd know if it had been opened – but I read the most recent ones between her and Sam, where she tells him she's lonely, hates her life, wishes she could live in Italy with him. The last email she sent was late last night, mentions some notes she saw in Mike's study about me. She goes on to say she thinks I might have something to do with the Peter Pan Killer, that it's fucking freaky because I look just like her.

The unread message is his reply. What did he say? What will she do?

I put the laptop back where I found it, leave and close the door, go along the corridor to my room. I lie down on my bed until it gets dark outside. Until the migraine subsides and no longer bears down on the back of my neck or pinches the top of my spine. I turn on my side, open my eyes, head hurts less now but when I look around my room, my heart hurts more. What will Phoebe do? What will happen to me? Where will I go?

I can't lie still any more so I go downstairs. Both Saskia and Mike are talking to Phoebe in the snug. I look for clues she's told them what she thinks she knows but nothing seems untoward.

'See, Mike, she's fine, there's no reason to stress about going out,' Saskia says.

Phoebe won't make eye contact with me, leaves the snug shortly after I arrive.

'Where are you guys going?' I ask.

'Sas and I have been invited to the Bowens' for dinner tonight but seeing as you're not feeling very well I thought we should stay home instead.'

'I feel better now after resting.'

Perhaps if they go out I could talk to Phoebe, reason with her, persuade her I'm different from you.

'I'm not sure we should go, you've had a lot to deal with recently,' Mike says.

'I'm fine, honestly, I'm going to catch up with some schoolwork.'

'I hope you'd tell us if you weren't, Milly, that's what we're here for.'

'Mike, she said she was okay, didn't she? Anyway, we cancelled last time, we really should go.'

Mike nods, says, looks like I've been out-voted. Once they have their coats on he delays their departure, a series of time-wasting tactics, sorts through the junk mail on the shelf by the door, uses his foot to rearrange the pile of shoes on the floor. Comments on how the porch could do with being re-tiled.

'Shall I quickly measure it now?' he says.

'No, we're already late, come on,' Saskia replies.

It's not maternal his instinct but he senses it, some kind of tension in the house. He makes a final attempt.

'What about Rosie then, she needs to go out.'

'One of the girls can do it,' Saskia replies.

'Are you sure you don't mind us going, Milly?'

'It's fine.'

'The number for the Bowens is on the blackboard, call us if you need anything, anything at all,' he says before they leave.

I don't know what to do. Whether I should go up to Phoebe's room, knock on the door. Ask her if I can talk to her about something, but I'm not sure what to say. I sit down on one of the sofas in the games room to think, Rosie at my feet. Her sharp ears hear it first, movement from above. She sits up, cocks her head, listens to Phoebe's footsteps coming down the stairs. She calls for Rosie, but the dog doesn't move. She calls again, this time more impatient. Forceful.

'She's in here with me,' I respond.

She doesn't answer straight away, must have thought I was elsewhere. Then she says without coming into the room, 'She needs to go out, Mum just texted me.'

Rosie gets up at the mention of going out, pads into the hallway towards Phoebe.

'For fuck's sake, I'll do it then.'

When she comes into the games room she ignores me, walks over to the patio door and opens it. Rosie follows her but won't go outside, sits down at the open door.

'Out, now.'

She still doesn't move so Phoebe grabs her collar, drags her out on to the patio. The security light goes on overhead. She stays outside with her even though she doesn't have a coat on and I know from the air filtering in, it's freezing. When Rosie's finished Phoebe brings her in, closes the door, her eyes trained on her phone. Mine, on her. It's now or never.

'Can I talk to you about something, Phoebe?'

She looks up from her phone but finds it hard to look directly at me, her eyes wandering all over the place.

'Depends.'

'I know we haven't really been getting on very well but I'd like that to change.'

'No point.'

'Why?'

'You won't be here for much longer.'

286

'I'd like to stay for as long as I can.'

'Not up to you, is it?'

I stand up, she looks at me, asks, 'What are you doing? One of my friends is coming over, he'll be here in a minute.'

She's scared. I don't want her to be. I want to tell her together we could run the world, a killer team, excuse the pun. She walks past me, gets to the doorway, and just before she leaves the room she says, 'Before you know it, Dad will have some other fucker in your room. It'll be like you never existed.'

32

The next day when I leave the school courtyard Phoebe's there with Clondine and Izzy. Clondine smiles but the other two turn away. How long have I got before smiles and ignoring turn into staring and pointing? That's her, can you believe it, the Peter Pan Killer's daughter.

When I get home both Mike and Saskia are there. Good timing, he says, we wanted to talk to you about something before the weekend begins. Saskia won't meet my eyes when we sit down, Mike offers to put the kettle on, neither of us replies.

'We wanted to tell you, Sas and I, that we're very proud of you, of what you've managed to do. There aren't many other teenagers I know that could have coped with such pressure, and in such a mature way, but now the trial's over we need to look forward and discuss what the future holds.'

Two days, that's all it's been since the verdict. Can't. Wait. To get rid of me.

'June and the social services team have been looking into a permanent placement for you. They think they might have found a potential family who live in the country near Oxford, lots of space and fields and two dogs, I believe. It's not confirmed yet, obviously you'll have to meet them and see how you get on, but it looks very promising. What do you think about the idea?'

'Sounds like I don't have a choice in the matter.'

'We don't want you to feel that way, we're just trying to work out what's best for you.'

'When am I leaving?'

'Milly, please don't be like that,' Mike says.

I cross my arms, feel for my scars. Turn my face away from them both.

'We'd really like you to have your birthday with us and finish the term at school, we'll have to work something out for the art prize exhibition.'

Too late, by that time everybody will know. The cat. Out of the bag.

'I feel so stupid.'

'What do you mean?' Mike asks.

'I thought you liked me.'

'We do,' Saskia replies. 'Very much.'

'Sas is right,' Mike says. 'But you staying here was never supposed to be a permanent arrangement, we spoke about this in hospital, remember?'

It was never supposed to be permanent because of Phoebe. Sugar and spice. And all things.

'Like we said, nothing is set in stone yet but we'll be looking at arranging a preliminary visit with the family in Oxford, perhaps even next weekend.'

The sooner the better, they all think.

It's the early hours of the morning and my head is clear for once. No battle raging inside me, pulling me this way and that. I suppose I've known for a while now that I don't belong here. Fit in. I've also known for a while that maybe there isn't anywhere for someone like me. If I'd known that before I left you, I might have stayed, nestled into a bosom that didn't necessarily give love but a familiar place to be. Birds of a feather.

I take the sock out of my underwear drawer, tip the pills I've been hiding into my hands, months of deceiving Mike. I walk into the bathroom, put them on the floor, bring my laptop too, slide the lock on the door, it can't be opened from the outside. I look at the pills, enough there I'm sure. I sit down, my laptop on my knees, a secret folder hidden in documents labelled:

You.

I reach for some of the pills, wash them down with a drink from a half-empty bottle of water I left by the sink. I watch the video clips of you arriving in a van. Windows, tinted black like Mike's car when I went to court too. The next clip is the last day of the trial. Verdict. Guilty times twelve. The crowd surged as the van transporting you left the courthouse, the press with their cameras held high. I take another mouthful, a mixture of blue and white pills, a few pink too. I press pause when the picture of you comes on screen. The room becomes furry after an hour or so, my body full of sand, slides down the wall a little. I feel like giggling, high from the drugs, but I don't remember how to, or the last time I did.

I take the rest of the pills, a good handful. Mainly pink, not to make the boys wink but so I don't have to think, any more. I take a gulp of water, mouth dry, a snail made of chalk meandering down my throat. I close the lid of the laptop, pull myself up on the side of the sink. This time I do want to look in the mirror, I want to see you before I go, but my hands slip off the side, the mirror melts. Bright spots of light in my eyes. Shooting stars. Make a wish, no point. I'm tired, so tired.

I climb into bed, no, I think it's the bath. The shower curtain moves in my hand, I need to cover myself quick, phone's at the ready, she takes pictures of me, remember. Fourteen tiles at the foot of the bath, I counted them the night before your trial began, when I couldn't sleep. My head rolls to my chest, a place of rest, a belly full of pills.

I'm pulled. My legs.

Grabbed from below.

Up eight. Up another four.
The door on the right.

Now I am dead, they'll find the things I hide.
The sketches of you taped back together.
Sick, they'll call me. Her mother's daughter.
There's other things too.
The first one by accident on my hands and knees cleaning the room.
A sugar cube on the floor. No. A milk tooth from a boy.
In my pocket it went.
After that I looked, searched. Pieces and bits, clothing, an item
from all nine, an obsession of mine smuggled out in my bag
the night of your arrest.
Why did I keep them?
Not treasure for the fairies, not under my pillow.
The answer, it was my way of caring for them.
Jayden. Ben. Olivia. Stuart. Kian. Alex. Sarah. Max. Daniel.
Nine little somethings I wanted to help.
You never knew I kept them.
Nobody did.

33

Tubes.

In me.

Lights.

Above me.

Dry throat, choking. A needle in the back of my hand, the shape of a butterfly. Wet on my face, a small stream. Tears. I don't want to cry, no point. Feel. Fear. Nothing to fear. Fear nothing. Fear everything.

Is anybody there?

Cold hands collide with my skin. Nudge. Turn. My eyes prised open with fingers. A blaze of light, a torch the size of a pen wages an assault on each pupil. A voice with an accent tells a story about a teenage overdose, stomach pumped. Attempted suicide. Multiple pills. Lucky.

Is that what you call it.

A language of numbers and letters, bloods and things. Things and blood. Discussed. A white coat, a clipboard in her arms, looks down at a chart. Pauses.

Increase sedation, the white coat says.

Pulled under again.

The next time I come round Mike's at my side. Air in my heart leaks, a balloon deflates. He's split open, his body bent over the bed. I can't speak, I've lost my voice, I've lost more than that. I squeeze his hand, he looks up.

'Milly, you're awake. Thank god you're awake.'

I try to reply, say sorry he couldn't fix me, I hate me, I'm bad on the inside.

'Don't try and talk, you need to rest,' he says.

He reaches above my head, presses a button. My pupils blink question marks, he reads them well, tells me a story. My story.

'You took an overdose, you didn't come down for breakfast so I came to check, the bathroom door was locked, we had to force it open. You've had your stomach pumped and you're heavily sedated still, everything's bound to be fuzzy for a while but you're going to be okay.'

The door to my room opens, I struggle to focus but the blonde hair gives her away.

'She's awake.'

'Yes, still spaced out on the meds, but awake.'

Saskia doesn't come to the bedside, stays back, but says, good, I'm glad, should we call someone?

'I have, one of the nurses should be here in a minute. Okay, Milly?'

I nod but I'm not sure I'll last. Eyelids, heavy. Mike, a speck. Smudged. The room is a boat. Seasick. A shadow, shiny and huge, a whale swims under, surfaces beside me, mouth open wide. I look inside. A mistake. I've made so many. They look back at me, their faces scared, hands reach out to me. I lean out of my boat as far as I can, I want to save them. A voice says 'No'. I've never heard him speak but I think it is god, the one I don't believe in. He laughs. Hard and relentless. The sea becomes wild, I can't get to them now. Nine, if I count. They hang their heads, they know what awaits, the whale closes its mouth, dives out of sight. I'm pulled back to the white, the room, too bright. A nurse speaks to Mike and Saskia, come with me please,

June's here. The next time I open my eyes Phoebe is there. Is she? Smile for the camera, dog-face. No, please don't, my voice a whisper, a foreigner to me. Too late. A flash in my face. You're the spit of your mother. I close my eyes, open them again straight away but she's not there, never was, my mind playing tricks on me.

There's a TV mounted on the wall, switched on but no volume, subtitles roll along the bottom of the screen. Headlines about the sinking of a ferry and just for a second I thought I saw your face. A machine to my left, previously a sleepy steady beat, now louder, attached to my heart, registers a reaction to you. I try to slow my breathing but the beeping gets faster, I close my eyes, pull me under again, please. I look back at the TV, the news is finished if it was ever on, a game show instead, contestants making up words.

I try to sit up, no strength in my arms. The conversation between June, Saskia and Mike. Where will I go? The new family won't want me now. We're not sure we can have that kind of person in our house, they'll say, isn't she better off staying where she is? Yes, I am, I realize that now. I want to stay. Room for us both, Phoebe and me. Please.

I turn back to the TV, your face fills the screen. Underneath, one word, flashing. Enlarged.

ESCAPED

You nod and smile, tell me you're coming for me. I hear someone screaming and realize it's me. I thrash in the bed, the butterfly in the back of my hand flies off, other tubes and wires too. The machine monitoring my heart emits an alarm, a dull continuous tone, the wire has come off, can't detect a heartbeat. Heartless. Can't. Find. My. Heart. A doctor runs in, calm down, calm down, he says, pushing my shoulders into the bed. Mike and Saskia enter the room next. The doctor shouts for somebody to get Olanzapine, 5mg IM.

'She's coming for me,' I hear myself say.

'Nobody's coming for you, Milly, you're safe.'

The nine little somethings watch from the corner of the room, their heads low, eyes moist, down-turned mouths.

A white coat.

A needle.

Sleep.

34

I'm transferred from the medical ward to the teenage psychiatric unit. It won't be for long Mike reasoned, a short focused admission to review your medication. No more than a week. He couldn't look me in the eyes when he said the word 'medication', as if it was his fault. Too blasé with handing them out, he thinks.

A nurse monitors my every move, they call it constant observation. A one on one. A clipboard hangs on the wall outside my room, every hour, on the hour, a tick on the page.

Toilet. Tick. Lunch. Tick. Alive. Tick.

Can I be left alone? No.

Can I go online? No.

Can I leave?

A slow shake of the head.

This time I play by the rules, I even take the pills they give me, maybe they help as I sleep for hours and don't see you once. June's been in a couple of times, said my placement with the Newmonts had been extended until after Christmas but following that I'll be moved into a new family. I ask her if Phoebe knows what happened. No. She thinks you had appendicitis, Mike told her there'd been a few complications but you'd be home soon.

How will she do it, I wonder. How will she tell everyone who I am?

The girl in the room next to mine visits too. She cradles a stuffed rabbit. Prozac meet Milly. Milly meet Prozac.

Why is he called Prozac, I asked her. She laughed, replied in a sing-song voice, my psychiatrist asks me that too. Yesterday the girl came into my room, stood at the side of my bed fondling the inner pink bits of the rabbit's ears, and said, I tell my psychiatrist I call bunny Prozac because he makes me feel better.

Josie, out of Milly's room please, one of the nurses said.

Quick, she said, give me your hand. She guided my finger through a hole in the rabbit's fur, another belly full of pills. But really it's because bunny likes Prozac too, she said, winked and pirouetted out of my room.

Little blue pills, gifts from the gods or the psychiatrists who prescribe them who think they are gods. I want to tell her to take them, do as they say, but I used to be her, squirrelling them away. Take them, don't take them, placebo spelt backwards is Obecalp. 10mg of Obecalp for the girl in room five please. I learnt fast at the first secure unit I stayed in, became wise to the language they used to try and fool us. Looking back, maybe I was the fool because after almost a week of staying here, taking my pills and talking to the nurses, I feel better.

Almost okay.

The discharge panel happened today. Mike and Saskia, June came too. A panel in psych is circular so you feel part of it, not like an interviewee. No uniforms either. Equals. Who decides who's mad, your words but I didn't want to hear them so I focused on telling the staff I felt safe. When they asked me, out of ten, how safe do you feel? A nine out of ten, I replied, I'm working on the last one. Smiles around the table, my attempt at a joke appreciated.

The overdose was attributed to delayed stress from the

trial and lack of sleep. No need to focus on it, let's move forward, the senior nurse said to Mike, this wasn't anybody's fault. Discharge granted, I get to go home, Friday 25 November, one week until I'm sixteen. I go to my room and pack up my things, no nurse at the door, I'm alive, no need to tick any more. A boy I've hardly seen enters my room, rushes at me, my back against the wall. His mouth is gluey with saliva, side effects from his pills, not a nice feeling when he's trying to get better. He tells me they're after me too, the men who come into his room at night. He whispers, looks behind him, don't let them in, he says. Even with the vulgar mess of his lips, the madness in his eyes, I fantasize about kissing him, telling him afterwards I'm dying. From what, he'd ask, did they do something to you? I don't know, I'd answer, something that happened a long time ago, I think. I want to tell him it won't be men that come for me in the night.

It'll be you.

How safe do you feel now?

One out of ten, maybe two.

35

Yesterday, Mike cancelled his Saturday clients and took the day off. He made everybody pancakes with bacon and maple syrup for breakfast, we all ate together and for once it went okay. Phoebe seemed happy, smiling. A glimmer of hope inside me, maybe she's decided to let go of the idea I'm something to do with you, or maybe she knows but feels sorry for me, wants to make it work between us. She and Saskia went out for the morning, a shopping trip, Mike looked so pleased. The simple things.

He supervises my medication closely now. The staff at the unit advised him to give me my pills with a warm drink, make me stay in the room long enough for the heat of the liquid to dissolve the drug into my bloodstream, and he does, which is fine. I want him to know he can trust me. I want to stay.

Once Saskia and Phoebe left we met for a session, he asked me what I'd like to talk about. I wanted to tell him I'd spent most of the week in the unit thinking about what Phoebe knows and what she's going to do about it, but instead I told him about being in the hospital room where my bed was a boat and how a whale swam underneath. I told him I'd imagined you on TV, the word 'escaped' on the screen. He explained it was the sedatives I was given, that they can create hallucinations. He also said he wanted me to come to him if I ever felt unsafe. That I was to stop bottling things up. We don't want you ending up back in hospital. Okay?

At the end of the session he handed me an envelope. I opened it, a get well card from Ms James. Mike explained he'd told everybody, not just Phoebe, that I had appendicitis, didn't feel it necessary to inform the school exactly what had happened given that the end of term was coming up. He asked if I thought I'd be ready to go back on Monday. Yes, I told him, I really like it at Wetherbridge, it's the best school I've been to. I'm also aware Miss Kemp knows, he said, Ms James emailed me, but you needn't be concerned, she won't tell anybody. No, I thought, but your daughter might.

Today, Mike and I decide to walk to the markets. On the way he tells me he's sent an email out about my birthday, arranged a tea at home next Saturday, there should be a good few folk popping by. I thank him but find myself lost in thoughts about what my sixteenth would have been like had I been with you.

We buy hot chocolate from one of the stalls and the lady who serves us asks me if I'm looking forward to Christmas. Yes, I tell her, but it's my birthday first. She looks at Mike, tries to guess my age. Looking at your dad I'd say you were seventeen. I smile, almost right, I'll be sixteen. I didn't care that she got it wrong because when she said 'looking at your dad', Mike didn't correct her. I go to smile at him but he's looking the other way, he didn't hear what she said.

After we get home I text Morgan to see if she's still coming over later. I wasn't allowed my phone in hospital, so by the time I was discharged there were loads of messages from her. She thinks it was my appendix too, and I'm hoping she won't ask to see the scar. I'm really looking forward to seeing her, making sure she's okay. The house is quiet for the rest of the afternoon. Phoebe's out, probably at Izzy's, and Saskia's having a lie-down. Mike's in his study, catching up with work, he said. Writing about me, maybe.

I try to sketch but I can't concentrate. I can't help thinking about Phoebe. It's not in her nature to let things go, it's not in her nature to try and understand. I wish I could go to her room, read her emails, but it's too risky with Mike around. She was happy at breakfast yesterday, smiling. It's not because I'm back, of course it's not, it's because she's thought of a plan.

I'm frightened. I miss the nurse ticking the form on the clipboard, Josie pirouetting around my room. I don't want to be on my own. Ground. Shaky. I want to tell Mike I'm worried Phoebe's found out but I'm not sure how to. I don't want him to know I've broken house rules, been into her room.

I don't know what I'm going to say to him but I go to his study anyway, he told me to come to him any time I needed to. I'm about to knock on the door, my hand mid-air, halfway to the wood, but I hear him talking to someone on the phone. I drop my arm down, turn my head so my ear's against the door, listen to the small talk. Plans for Christmas and New Year, then I hear him talking about me.

'I think you're right, June, it's time for Phoebe to come first, no question about that. I'm sorry we've changed our minds, but now that Milly's back I realize it's too much having both of them here and, to be honest, supporting her through the trial and with what happened recently, it's taken its toll on me. On all of us. I could use a bit of normality again.'

He pauses, as June responds.

'Yes, agreed, it feels too early to tell her, too soon after the overdose, but I'm sure she'll be fine when I do. I'll be gentle.'

I back away from the door. I don't feel like telling him I'm scared any more. He told me to stop bottling things up, but how can I talk to someone who I know doesn't want me here.

When Morgan arrives on my balcony the sight of her moves me. Is home a place or is it a person? We sit on the bed, she asks me how I'm feeling but not to see the scar. I ask her how she is too, she was injured the last time I saw her, the swelling around her mouth gone, the scrape on her forehead healed.

'You know how your favourite book's *Peter Pan*, Mil?'

'Yeah?'

'Well, it's also my sister's favourite movie. We watched the DVD last week and you know how Peter gets something for Wendy to say thanks? Well, I got you something.'

She takes it out of her pocket, hands it to me. It's a small gold locket similar to the ones I've seen at the antique stalls in the market. I open it, no pictures inside.

'I thought maybe one day you could put my picture in one side and yours in the other.'

Both of us smile and I realize how much she means to me and that I don't have to hurt her to keep her safe. She's doing okay as she is. She lies down on the bed, I ask if I can sketch her. I want to start a new series of portraits, one where I don't have to smudge the faces.

36

I found my first couple of days back at school difficult, the noise in the canteen louder, the collisions in the corridors harder. The perpetual fear of Phoebe spreading the word. I've tried my best to stay out of her way, hoping as if by magic she'll forget who I am. Who she thinks I am. The waiting is worse – not knowing why she hasn't told anybody yet.

When school ends today I go down to the locker room to collect my stuff and she's there with Marie, who asks her to go to Starbucks. Phoebe says no, there's some stuff she needs to do at home.

'I'll walk out with you though if you give me a minute, I just need to read this email.'

She smiles as she looks at the screen of her phone.

'Who's it from?' Marie asks.

'Nobody,' she replies, glancing over at me. 'It's just about something I've got planned for tomorrow.'

Couldn't put Humpty together again.

On the way up to the Great Hall I send Mike a message, remind him I'll be set-building for the play until seven. He replies saying not to worry, both he and Saskia will be at his office celebrating the refurb completion, they'll be back a similar time to me. Keeping busy is the trick, I focus on painting and building, and halfway through the evening I offer to go to the shop just by school, buy snacks for everybody, a much-needed sugar hit. I realize when we finish just after seven, with a good bit of the set built, I enjoyed it, a welcome distraction.

I walk out with MK, tell her I've started a new series of portraits. She's pleased, time to move on, she says. Yes, I agree. It is.

'Will you be all right getting home?' she asks.

'Fine thanks, I live super close.'

'Okey-doke. See you tomorrow, Milly.'

'Bye.'

I'm halfway home when my phone rings. Mike's name flashing on the screen and when I answer he says, 'Where the hell are you?'

'I'm just walking home, I've been –'

'You are not to come home, do you hear me?'

His voice is forced, strained. So different from normal.

'Go next door to Valerie's and stay there until I say so.'

'Mike, you're scaring me, what's happened?'

'Do as I say. Do not come home, do you hear me?'

'Yes.'

As I approach the house it looks normal. I don't want to go to Valerie's but she's waiting for me on the road, hurries me inside to hers.

'What's going on?' I ask her. 'Mike scared me.'

'We're not really sure at the moment but it'll be okay. Come on in, out of the cold.'

Every time I've heard those words – it'll be okay – it never has been.

It doesn't take long. I hear sirens first, screaming to a halt outside our house. Valerie takes me into the living room overlooking the garden, not the street, asks me if I'd like something to eat or drink.

'I want to go home, I want to know what's happened.'

308

'Not just now, sweetheart.'

I don't get to go home for almost two hours. Valerie puts the TV on, does her best to look normal. Relaxed. But when David, her husband, comes home I can tell from the looks they exchange. News is bad. Bad news. The doorbell goes, David answers it, I hear him talking to Mike, brings him into the room. When I see him I burst into tears because his shirt is stained, all over the front, and I know what kind of stain makes that colour. He looks down and says in a monotone voice, 'I should have changed, I didn't think.'

His voice is slow, his face terrorized. Aged. He'll see red too now, a member of the same club as me.

'Valerie, perhaps we should give them a minute,' David suggests.

'Of course, take as long as you need.'

They close the door behind them, the atmosphere in the room serious. Charged. Mike sits next to me. I notice his hands are shaking. Normality, that's what he'd been hoping for, the conversation with June.

'I'm frightened, Mike, what's going on? Please tell me.'

He can't get the words out, keeps starting and stopping. Mouth. Struggling to release the ugly it knows it has to. Finally, he says, 'An accident, a terrible accident.'

He covers his face with his hands, also stained, all over his fingers. I want to reach out and touch him but I don't want any of it on my skin.

'What do you mean?'

He doesn't answer initially, shakes his head, looks down at the rug under our feet. Disbelief. I've seen it before in the detective I gave my first statement to. Mike takes his hands away from his face but immediately brings one back up to cover his mouth after saying her name. Hyperventilating. He finds it easy to calm other people down, it's his job, but when it comes to himself he's lost.

'What sort of accident? Is she okay?'

Breath laboured, hand reaches up at the tie he's wearing. Tries to pull it loose. It won't help I want to tell him, nothing will.

'No, not okay,' he says.

But he doesn't say she's dead, so much red on his shirt though. So much red.

'What do you mean not okay? Can I see her? I want to see if she's all right.'

He pulls at his hair, pulls at his shirt, hands won't stay still, can still feel the shape of her body. He begins to rock, mutters to himself.

'Mike, please, talk to me.'

'She's gone, the paramedics have taken her away, the police are at the house.'

'Gone where?'

He turns to look at me, grabs my knees. Hands like claws. The 'don't touch Milly' rule gone out the window. I want to move away, close my eyes. I don't want to see the look in his when he says what I think he's going to say next.

'She's dead, Milly, my Phoebs is dead.'

Then he starts to cry, removes his hands from my legs, hugs himself. Arms crossed over his chest, he begins to rock again.

'I don't understand, I saw her at school just after the bell went.'

He stands up suddenly. Movement to diffuse the bad feelings inside, it helps me too. Sometimes. He walks to the fireplace, back again. Mumbling and muttering as he does. He paces for what feels like for ever then stops, looks at me, as if he's just remembered somebody else is in the room with him. He comes over, kneels on the floor in front of me, psychologist's hat inching back on. Solid ground. Knows how to play that role, it's easier, more comfortable than being on the wrong side of grief.

'I'm sorry, Milly,' he says, 'I'm sorry.'

'Why are you saying sorry?'

'You've already had so much to deal with.'

Then he breaks down, huge racking sobs, every breath an effort. I start to cry again too, his pain flooding the space around me. I try to tell him it'll be okay, somehow it'll be okay. I reach out, place my hand on his head. I think it helps as he stops crying so hard, sits back on his heels and begins to massage each side of his temples, runs his fingers through his hair, two, three times. Big breaths, that's what he takes now, in through his nose, out through his mouth.

'What happened?' I ask him.

'We think she fell, the police are investigating now.'

'Fell?'

'I can't go over the details, Milly. Please. Not now.'

'Where's Saskia?'

In hell, I think his answer would be if he could say it out loud, if he could bring himself to. I smell whisky on his breath when he speaks. He said he couldn't go over the details but he can't help it, they're playing on a loop, a broken record inside his head. Her phone was on the floor next to her, he keeps saying. I told her not to sit up there, one day she'd fall. She never listened though, did she. She never bloody listened. He begins to cry again, covers his face.

'It's not your fault, Mike.'

311

I hear the doorbell ring, voices again. A gentle knock at the door. Valerie comes into the room, says, sorry, but the police want to talk to you, they say you can go home if you like. Mike nods, uses both hands to pull himself up on the sofa, legs not to be trusted. Valerie leaves, says she'll wait in the hallway.

'We should go,' he says.

'I'm scared, what will I see?'

'You won't see anything. There's a tarpaulin over where she —'

He walks over to the window, leans his hand against the glass, looks into the garden, composes himself. Tries to. He turns to face me, says, we have to go. When we leave the room Valerie and David are waiting outside, they both say how sorry they are and if there's anything they can do, just to call, no matter what time of day. Mike nods.

The first thing I see in the driveway is two police cars, no ambulance, already gone Mike said. When we get to the front door I don't want to go in.

'I'm not sure I can, Mike.'

'We have to. I'll be with you the whole time.'

A group of uniformed officers are standing in the entrance hallway. Mike introduces me as his foster daughter. One of them nods, and says Steve's in the kitchen waiting. The floor, new tiles will be needed. I hold on to Mike as we pass.

'You're okay,' he says, his hand on my back. I ask again where Saskia is.

'The ambulance crew gave her an injection, something to calm her down, she's in our bedroom.'

Another officer is seated at the table, stands up as we walk in.

'You must be Milly. Is it okay if I ask you some questions? I understand this must be a terrible shock for you.'

'Can I stay with her?' Mike asks.

'Of course, it won't take long, routine stuff really. Please, sit down.'

He opens the notepad in front of him, takes the lid off a biro.

'Can you tell me the last time you saw Phoebe?'

'At school, at the end, it would have been about four o'clock.'

'How did she seem to you?'

'Normal, I guess. She was on her phone.'

'Do you know who to?'

'No, she was reading an email. Seemed excited about something.'

He makes a note in his pad.

'And did she tell you what she was excited about?'

'No.'

'And she said she was going straight home?'

'I think so, yeah, she said she had some stuff to do.'

'Was anything else said between the two of you?'

'Not really no, I had a meeting to go to. I'm helping design the set for our play.'

'And that's where you've been this evening?' he asks.

'Yes, there's about fifteen of us and one of the teachers, Miss Kemp.'

Another note in his pad.

'What time did you leave school?'

'I walked out with my teacher, just after seven, that's when Mike called me.'

The officer looks at Mike, he nods to confirm what I've said is correct, his face looking older by the minute. I can tell it's over when the officer closes his notebook, the lid back on his biro. The detail of people.

'I'm sorry for your loss. I think we're done here,' he says.

He pauses a few seconds, a polite response to what he sees, awake in his training, he was. As he stands, his chair scrapes across the tiles. Mike flinches, every noise and sensation heightened now.

'Will you be staying here tonight?' he asks.

'Possibly, depending on how my wife is. They gave her an injection.'

'Would you like me to arrange a clean-up team to come in? It'll not be a perfect job at this time of day but enough to get you through the night.'

'If you could, thank you,' Mike replies.

I shield my eyes as I pass the tarpaulin. Mike tells me to stay in my room until he says otherwise.

'If Saskia's awake we'll move into a hotel tonight, if not, first thing tomorrow.'

Three messages on my phone from Morgan asking if I'm okay and what's with the police cars at the house. I text her, tell her I'm fine but Phoebe's not, she's dead, she fell off the banister. Fuck, she replies instantly, she was well mean but I wouldn't wish that on anyone, accidents are the worst.

Yes, I reply.

The worst.

37

We've been living in a hotel for the past week, Rosie in kennels. The house no longer felt like home, the marble in the hallway needed lifting. Replaced. The area, deep cleaned again. I can't help imagining how Mike and Saskia would have reacted when they found Phoebe's body. Saskia. Dropped to her knees I bet, screaming, Mike there by her side. Footsteps. Urgent. He would have run to Phoebe's body, checked for a pulse, that's why his hands and his shirt were stained. He'd have crumpled on to the floor, gathered her body into his. Saskia, mute, after the shock set in.

I worry for them both, the spotlight on their grief shines twenty-four seven. Mike, going through the motions, moving more slowly than usual, each step reminds him of what he saw. He's the keeper of the pills, both Saskia, if she makes it out of bed, and I line up in the mornings. She takes whatever he gives, her hand outstretched for more. She slept all day, Mike told me when I returned from my first day back at school, a sense of structure, normality, enforced on me. I thought I'd be glad to escape but I just want to be with them. Mike feels it too, says it helps when I come back each day.

During the night, through the wall, I hear Saskia weep, their room in the hotel next to mine, a sad continuous noise, childlike. Grief does that, it ages with its horror yet diminishes too, back to a state where we want to be coddled and protected from the world. Yesterday we were given the all-clear to return home. Not so long ago I would have gone straight to my room, taken out a sketch of you, traced the outline of your face, but I don't. I spend as much time as I can with Mike, providing warm drinks, snacks, taking care of Rosie. Being useful. Sevita has been given time off, as much as she needs. Devastated Mike said she was when he phoned her the day after it happened. Phoebe and she were so close, he said.

I heard him crying on the phone yesterday, talking to his dad in South Africa, too elderly to travel, won't make the memorial being held in the Great Hall at school today. Saskia's seen nobody, calls nobody, her parents died when she was in her twenties, no siblings. Mike's been rescuing girls for years.

Yesterday a steady stream came to the house. Hushed voices, cards, flowers. Friends. Enemies. Frenemies. There's been a marked change towards me at school as if Phoebe's death has evaporated a force field of isolation erected by her around me. Clondine hugged me the first time she saw me, cried into my neck, I went to the toilets afterwards, washed her tears off my skin.

Today when we arrive in the Great Hall we're met with a sea of pink, Phoebe's favourite colour. Hats, skirts, a feather boa, one big, pink sorority gathering. Hundreds of eyes on us as we walk to the front. I managed in court but this crowd feels worse, somehow.

Ms James talks about Phoebe's achievements and the promise she held for the future, successful at whatever she'd have chosen. A wave of sobs and nose-blowing fills the hall. Girls lean into each other, some genuinely sad, others enjoying the drama such as teenage girls do. Clondine next, dedicates a poem to Phoebe. The last two lines, do not stand at my grave and cry, I am not there, I did not die.

Mike goes on to the stage, thanks the school for their support. I slide into his chair so I'm next to Saskia. Eyes. Glassy like a doll. Distant. Lost. Chemicals take her there. Izzy ends the service by playing guitar and singing 'Somewhere Over the Rainbow'. Drinks are served in the library afterwards. Miss Kemp comes over, offers her condolences, the skin on her hands still dry. People mill in the spaces around the three of us, hands touch my back, my shoulders and my arms. I do my best not to flinch. Such a terrible accident they say, yes, I reply. Terrible.

Just before we leave, Izzy's mum approaches us, small and French. Toxic. Now I know where her daughter gets it from.

'What good can come from this?' she says. 'A mindless tragedy.'

Mike nods, she turns to look at me.

'Have you enjoyed your time at Wetherbridge?'

Enjoyed. The past tense.

'I heard you'll be moving on somewhere new soon, Sas told me before this happened.'

Saskia says nothing, cat's got her tongue, or it's the chemicals she swallows every day.

'Anyway,' she says, '*quelle bonne nouvelle*. What wonderful news.'

She kisses Mike and Saskia, ignores me. When she's gone, Mike apologizes. I nod, try to look brave, but all around me tiny angels raise tiny trumpets, for Phoebe, not me.

★

After the school memorial Mike and Saskia went on to Phoebe's funeral. A small service, family and close friends. Mike left me at Valerie's, said it was better if I didn't come, he and Saskia needed time to say goodbye. I said I understood but I felt disappointed he still doesn't view me as family and I know it's selfish to be thinking like that but I can't help it. Like a carrot being dangled. Room for me now.

You came to me, in the middle of the night, the first visit in weeks. You said it was time. Time for what, I asked. You didn't reply but shed your skin before you left, a scaly outline under my pillow, so real I check for it now.

I'm not able to sleep, find myself opening the door to Phoebe's room. Her smell remains strong, sweet and inviting. I close the door behind me. Her room is as she left it, school bag and folders dumped on the floor, a copy of *Lord of the Flies* on the bedside table. In time Mike and Saskia will go through her belongings, dismantle her life. I open the drawer in her desk but her laptop's not there, I check in the bottom of the wardrobe and inside her bag. She might have left it at school but she hardly ever took it. I don't like the fact it's not here, I don't like the way it makes me feel.

38

My birthday tea was cancelled, it was supposed to be last weekend but we were staying in the hotel. So we're having it today instead, the Saturday before term ends, a quiet dinner, no guests, Mike said. Just the three of us. When I go down to the kitchen there's a present on the table addressed to me. I open it. It's a watch with a message inscribed on the back: HAPPY 16TH WITH LOVE M & S. The feeling it gave me. Like I belong.

When Mike comes in I notice the way he moves, still much slower than he used to before Phoebe's accident. Simple tasks like filling the kettle require more effort, the exhaustion of being alive when someone you love isn't. His shirt is done up wrong but I don't have the heart to tell him so I take the kettle from his hands and ask him to sit down. He does without protest.

I've hardly seen Saskia but when I do her eyelids are red, swollen, like living up close with one of the mothers you stole from. How they must have felt knowing they'd never see or hold their child again. Once I've made a pot of tea, I ask Mike if I can take her a cup.

'You can try,' he says. 'She's going to make an effort for today.'

I take the tea up to her room, knock on the door, no response. I knock again, this time she says, come in. The room's dark, a small amount of natural light creeping in from the window in the bathroom. The air is still. Dusty.

She's thinner in frame, doesn't see Benji any more, doesn't see anybody.

'I made you some tea.'

She nods but doesn't move from where she's sat on the edge of the bed.

'Shall I leave it here for you?'

She nods again, I place it on the dressing table, her eyes fill up with tears. Kindness when you're wounded hurts more.

'Sorry, I shouldn't have disturbed you.'

She wipes the tears away, shakes her head.

'The house is so quiet without her. Silly really, all I ever wanted was peace and now she's gone all I want is her.'

I don't say anything, not yet. I've been reading articles on the internet on what to do, how to help people when they're grieving. Little things like hot food on the table, emptying the bins. Being visible but not intrusive, letting them talk if they want to.

'I miss her, even the times she hated me. Don't say she didn't, we all know I'm not the best mother.'

Her fingers trace the edges of the name necklace. Gold. She smiles a little, a sad smile. A realization of sorts. She yanks hard on the chain, it breaks, dangles from her finger-tips before dropping to the floor.

'I never got it right with Phoebe, any of it.'

I sit next to her on the bed, take one of her hands in mine, tell her I think she did get it right, that she's a good mum – I remind her of the crystal she bought me. She cries, leans her body against my shoulder. We sit like that for a while. I feel her tears soaking through the cotton of my T-shirt. I don't like it but I stay, hoping these are the moments she and Mike will remember when decisions are made about where I might go.

'I should shower,' she says.

I nod and as I leave I remind her to drink the tea. When Mike sees me, he asks me how she is.

'She's getting up, she's going to have a shower.'

'Well done, you had better luck than me.'

'I want to do anything I can to help.'

'And you are, you've been keeping us going. If it was just me and Sas I'm not sure where we'd be.'

Tiny trumpets raised in salute, this time for me.

A couple of hours later a knock on my bedroom door. Saskia, doing her best. In her hands she carries a bag. Cosmetic.

'I'd like to do your make-up, would that be okay?'

I nod, we sit down together on the bed, she talks as she sweeps. Powder and bronze. Each time her wrist passes near to my nose I'm hit with a scent so feminine extra blush arrives on my face. It's hardly touch what she does to me now but it's intimate. Eye contact this close, still uncomfortable for me.

'Phoebe never let me do her make-up, said I didn't do it right, am I doing yours right?'

I nod, and say, of course, you're doing a great job, though I have no idea if it's true.

'You're very beautiful, Milly, I don't think you know that.'

She talks and talks, tells me Phoebe was a mistake, she'd had the flu and forgotten to take her contraceptive pill for a few days. A shock. A difficult baby, not easy to soothe.

I'm tempted to ask her about Benji — a secret when handled carefully can be useful — gives a person leverage. Gives me leverage if Saskia thinks we're bonding, keeping each other's secrets, but for once, she's ahead of me.

'I'd like us to spend more time together, Milly. Would you like that?'

'Yes, very much, but I might be leaving soon.'

'Mike and I have been talking, the house is already so empty.'

'Does that mean I –'

'What?'

'It doesn't matter, it's just I really like it here with you guys.'

She nods and smiles a little, says, 'Mike said you bought a dress, shall I help you into it?'

'No, thank you.'

I ask her to get a camera, I'd like a photo of me and her if it's okay.

My dress. Black, long-sleeved velvet, a skater-style skirt attached, puffs out a bit, lands on my knees. I wear tights and a pair of black heeled boots I bought with my allowance from Topshop similar to the ones I've seen the other girls wear. I wish I could finish the outfit with my gold name necklace but I know it's the wrong thing to do so I put on the necklace Morgan bought me instead and the watch from Mike and Saskia, and I can't help but feel loved.

She comes back with the camera, Mike at her side. She's barefoot, childlike. More like a sister than a mother.

'Stunning,' Mike says.

He puts his arm round Saskia's waist and even though she moves away from him, I know they will fuck tonight. A new beginning.

For my birthday meal we eat Chinese in the kitchen. Mike says I look too fancy for takeaway, the first joke I've heard him attempt since Phoebe's death. Sorry we haven't gone out for dinner, he said, but we can't really face it at the moment.

There's a fortune cookie for each of us but neither Mike nor Saskia want to open theirs. I save mine for later, to open alone when we're finished. Mike says he got an email from Joe's dad asking if Joe could see me some time. Saskia nods, says, he's a nice boy, I've met him before.

'Is that okay with you, Milly?'

'Yeah.'

I imagine him taking me to the cinema, his freckles turning pink as he kisses me goodnight, but then I remember what kisses lead to and I don't like the thought very much any more.

I offer to clear up, tell Mike and Saskia to go and relax in the snug. I look in as I pass, they're sitting on the same sofa. Saskia's body is turned, her back against the arm, her feet tucked down the gap between the cushions in the middle. Mike sits beside her, his hand on her shin.

'We should light the fire soon, Sas, we usually do in December.'

'I can't believe it's December already,' she replies.

They stare at the unlit fire, both thinking about the same thing, the same person. I leave them like that, go up to my room and call Morgan. I haven't seen her much since Phoebe's accident, I've been focusing on Mike and Saskia, on filling their void and making friends at school. I'm doing okay, I think. Offering to help fundraise for the senior common room was a wise move, instantly elevated me. A phoenix. Messy. But rising.

When she answers she tells me she has to be quiet, her little sister's asleep next to her, asks me what I've been up to. Not much, I tell her, just school and helping out at

323

home. I miss you, Mil, she says, can you tell me a story. Okay, close your eyes first though. I tell her the names of the stars, the planets. There's water on Mars. I tell her about the catacombs in Paris, a cemetery of skulls underground. Sounds amazing, she says, I'd like to go, maybe we can go one day. Maybe, yes. We arrange to see each other next weekend and after I hang up I open the fortune cookie. The message reads: IF YOU HAVE SOMETHING GOOD IN YOUR LIFE, DON'T LET IT GO.

I look at the watch on my wrist and think, I don't plan to, whatever it takes.

39

We receive a standing ovation for our performance of *Lord of the Flies*. I played Phoebe's part, the narrator, am pushed forward by the girls at the end of the show. You were amazing, take another bow, go on. I look out into the audience, see Mike and Saskia clapping. Mike's looking at me strangely, doesn't take his eyes off me. Doesn't smile either.

After the play's over I offer to help tidy away the props. Clondine and I leave at the same time. She stops and looks up at the sky.

'It's so sad.'

'What is?'

'It's the Christmas dance this Friday, it was Phoebe's favourite. She loved all the fancy dresses and wearing Saskia's fur.'

I say it's sad too, because it is.

Walking home, I look on my phone at the BBC news page. Nothing about you for weeks but this evening, a headline. Our house is to be demolished, a community garden planted. Nine trees. You don't come to me in my bed any more, you shed your skin. 'It's time,' you said. I understand now what you meant, that I didn't need you any more. A mixture of happy and sad. Mostly I'm coming to terms with the things I've done. I did them to be good, I promise, even though they were bad.

I've been practising what to say, in case you ever come back.

This is what I'd say.

I never asked for a mother who wolf-whistled at me, who laughed in my face when I tried to say no. I'd tell you, you were wrong when you used to stand behind me at the mirror in your bedroom and say nobody will ever love me but you, because I think Mike and Saskia might grow to. I'd tell you, you were right, my insides do look different to everybody else's.

A curious, twisted shape.

The shape you made me. The shape I'm learning to live with.

The night of your arrest, I nodded at you. You knew what I meant. I was telling you I was leaving you. I was ready. But you weren't, were you? You never liked it when a game ended, you always wanted to keep playing. The game you made me play, going to court, more public than we'd ever done before. A last fire of the gun, a parade of how well you'd taught me. It wasn't a walk in the park, no, nor was it checkmate. It was like turning my face to the sun. Blinding. No shade.

Your voice, to me, was a morphine drip. Sullied, not able to provide relief and comfort, but fear and temptation instead. I'm glad I no longer hear you or see you in places I know you can't be, like standing at the bus stop by school.

The things you did, the things you made me do, broke my heart.

You broke my heart.

You broke my.

You broke.

You.

And me.

Because of that, I have secrets, so many secrets.

I am not who I say I am.
Folie à deux – a madness shared by two.
Deny.
Manipulate.
Lie.
Mummy, I thought I could choose.
It turns out, I'm just like you.

Only better.

Being good doesn't interest me any more.

Not

    Getting

        Caught

            Does

40

I know something's wrong as soon as I open the front door. It's where Mike's standing, in the middle of the tiles where she landed. Why is he standing there when for the past week or so he hasn't been able to look at them, never mind stand on them.

'I need you to come to the study. Right now,' he says.

He doesn't ask me to sit down when we get there, he stands closer to me than normal, looks into my eyes. I don't think he likes what he sees because he walks away, sits down at his desk, mutters to himself. There's a bottle of whisky, over a third empty, a glass on his desk. He drains the measure already poured, pours another one right away. I sit down in silence on the armchair that has become mine over the past few months. And wait.

His words, when they come, hurt me.

'I was warned about you. People said I was stupid. Reckless even. Having you here would only cause trouble, but I didn't listen, I thought I could handle it.'

The piranhas are back. The fortune fish too, a new trial beginning.

'I thought I knew everything about you — maybe not everything, but most things. I thought you trusted me. I trusted you, I took you in for god's sake.'

'I do trust you, Mike.'

His fist crashes down on his desk, I jump. It's nothing compared to what you used to do but from Mike, gentle, understanding Mike, it feels savage. Brutal. He's angry with me. His head's starting to clear, grief is a fog, a mist. Hangs low, obscures the landscape. Obscures what's really there.

'Don't lie to me,' he says. 'If you trusted me, you would have told me.'

'Told you what?'

He pauses, downs a mouthful of whisky, arches his fingers on the desk. Twin tarantulas, ready to pounce.

'In our sessions, the things you said. Jumbled. Inconsistent. You were so hard to guide. You hated me asking you about it, tried hard not to say his name, but I knew something about the night Daniel died troubled you more than I thought it should. But when I asked you, kept asking you, the story was the same and I believed you. I wanted to at some level, you'd been through so much, but now I'm not sure any more. I'm not sure of anything.'

His fingers relax on the desk, more pianist than spider. Whisky is also a mist, one that confuses the mind until you're not sure what to believe any more. Drink some more, please, Mike.

'What you told the court, about what happened that night, was it true, Milly? Did your mother kill Daniel? Did she?'

'Why do you think I'm lying?'

'Because you do, don't you? You lie. You lied to me, didn't you? You lied to me about Phoebe when you said you were getting on fine.'

'We were.'

He swipes a glass paperweight off his desk, it collides with the wall, doesn't break, leaves a dent in the paintwork, lands on the ground with a thud.

'You're scaring me, Mike.'

'Well you scare me, do you know that?'

There it is. The truth. His. He feels the same about me as everyone else does. As I do about myself. I lower my gaze.

'I'm sorry, that was unnecessary, Milly.'

He drinks another whisky, adjusts the photo frame that sits on the right-hand side of his desk. I felt jealous and lonely when I first saw the pictures in the frame. A collage of Phoebe, all different ages. Blonde and perfect and beautiful, not contaminated like me. He shakes his head, smiles at his daughter. Not fondly, but with regret perhaps. Regret about what? She's gone but she's everywhere still, in the spaces and gaps that are supposed to be mine now.

The phone on his desk rings, he looks over at it but doesn't pick it up.

'It'll be June,' he says. 'I called her while I was waiting for you to come back but she didn't answer. She'll know something's up though, I wouldn't normally call this late.'

'Why did you?'

'I'm writing a book about you, did you know that? No. Well, I am. It was all I was able to think about. How stupid and arrogant of me.'

He doesn't tell me why he called June but I can feel the place in this family I've been carving, manipulating, since Phoebe's death, start to dissolve in front of me. Quicksand. Sinking. Me.

'You can stop pretending now, Milly. I know.'

And all the king's horses and all the king's men.

'It had been going on for months, hadn't it? Facebook, the school forum. Text messages. The police returned Phoebe's phone yesterday. She'd been bullying you for months, hadn't she?'

I know what he's thinking, that all roads lead to me.

'Why didn't you tell me? Christ, we spent enough time together.'

'I didn't want to worry you or cause any trouble. I thought Phoebe and I might become friends – sisters, even.'

He opens one of the drawers in his desk, removes something, looks down at it then lifts it up and places it in front of him.

Phoebe's laptop, Mike had it.

'She didn't think I knew,' he says.

'Knew what?'

'About Sam.'

'Sam who?'

'You're telling me you didn't know, hadn't heard anything about it at school?'

'No, nothing.'

He asks me if I'm lying. I don't answer because I am but only because I'm too scared to tell the truth. The flashes of what could be a new life for me here in this house stop me. So close. If I can just ride this next storm, if I can persuade him.

'His dad and I go way back. We studied together years ago, stayed in touch when they moved to Italy, we saw them this summer. We'd all been having a bit of a laugh about it behind their backs, a long-distance romance. Sam's mum had seen some of the emails but not all of them. Not the ones where Phoebe told him her suspicions about you.'

'But I thought she didn't know about me?'

'Well she did,' he replies.

His fists clench, open. Clench. He reaches for the bottle of whisky, pours a measure, drains it again but doesn't pour another. I wish he would, his edges and ability to reason are starting to soften with the warmth of the alcohol, I can see it.

'She came to me a while ago, said she'd seen some notes about you in my study while looking for a book. I tried to tell her it wasn't true but she got so upset, said I was always putting my patients first. I couldn't lie to her any more, I didn't want to, so I told her but we agreed she wouldn't say anything and she didn't, not to anyone at school anyway, only to Sam.'

'I'm sorry, Mike.'

'You've said that a lot since I've known you. What exactly is it you're sorry for?'

He doesn't wait for me to answer, the conversation he's having is more with himself than me. He's trying to put things in the right place in his head. Tidy up, file them away. Reassure himself he didn't get it wrong, so horribly wrong.

'She had plans to expose you, you know. It's there, written in an email to Sam, the last one she sent after school on the day she died. She'd bought a pay-as-you-go phone, was going to send out anonymous text messages, tell everybody who you were. Goddamn it, how did I miss how unhappy she was?'

'It's not your fault, Mike.'

Small nods of his head, but somehow it feels like it is, he replies. He stares at Phoebe's laptop, looks at the photo frame of her again. I start to cry, it hurts me to see it up close. The damage I've caused, a terrorist in his family, shape-shifting each time.

When he notices I'm crying, he says, 'You're usually very good at hiding your feelings.'

'What do you mean?'

'The bullying must have hurt, made you upset. Angry.

Yet you never showed it. I knew you and Phoebe weren't close but I never noticed any major animosity, any major concerns.'

He's lying to himself. He noticed, in the same way he notices Saskia swimming through the motions. Drunk, high, depressed. Repeat. Drunk, high, depressed. His emerald city at home, fucked up. If he was honest with himself, if he was brave enough, he'd admit that it suited him not to notice, not to acknowledge the tension between Phoebe and me. He wanted me here, needed me. Access to my mind, a golden opportunity, one that would likely never come around again. Female killers, like I said, are rare.

'We hid it from you, both of us.'

'I should have been able to see it. So bloody absorbed with work, and –'

'Writing about me.'

He nods, replies, yes, but at what cost.

'Is that why you feel bad, you feel like you should have spent less time with me and more with Phoebe?'

He leans back in his chair, pushes his body against the leather. I know how it feels when you don't want to talk about things but you're still being asked. Nobody wants to talk about the things they feel guilty about.

'Phoebe loved you so much, Mike. I could see that.'

He shakes his head, his turn for the tears to come.

'She did, Clondine told me the night of Matty's party at half-term that Phoebe idolized you, thought you were the best dad in the world.'

'How could I have been, I was too busy, too busy involving myself with other people's problems.'

'That's what she loved about you. The fact you care and try to help.'

My words anoint, rub soothing oil and balm into his loss, his guilt. I can see the game beginning to change in front of my eyes. I stand up, walk over to his desk, pour him another whisky. Drink it, I tell him, it'll help. He does, he's used to me helping. I've worked hard recently to make it so him and Saskia couldn't be without me. Wouldn't want to be. He watches me as I sit back down. I pick up the blue velvet cushion he placed on the chair in our first session together. I hold it, pull it into my chest. It'll trigger a response, remind him I'm still a child, someone who needs love and care. Guidance. It'll activate his desire, his need to be needed. A hero complex hidden underneath expensive shirts. Pride. A long way to fall if you get things like me wrong.

'I've said some things I shouldn't have, Milly. I'm sorry. I thought I'd worked everything out, I thought I knew.'

Knew what? Why did he call June?

'Miss Kemp told me tonight she was so thankful for your help with the set design, she said you'd worked so hard at the last meeting, even went out and bought snacks for everybody. I hadn't been able to think clearly since Phoebe's death until today.'

'You're tired, Mike, from trying to look after everyone.'

'That's why I called June, I wanted to speak to her about something. I was so clear about it then but now I don't know. I think I was looking for someone to blame and I'm ashamed to admit that that person was you.'

He runs his finger round the rim of the glass, pauses, then looks up at me.

'I asked Miss Kemp what time you went out to get the snacks. She wasn't sure, so much going on, but said you were only gone for five minutes or so.'

How would she know, chaotic keeper of the time.

'Were you?' he asks.

'Was I what?'

He asks the next question quietly. Slowly.

'Were you only gone for five or so minutes?'

Usually it's the truth he wants to hear but this time the road doesn't only lead to me, it leads to him. Too engrossed and obsessed with wondering about me, writing about me. The book has a different ending now, one he doesn't want to write. He didn't just invite me in for tea, he invited me to live with him, with his family. He'd never recover personally or professionally if he felt, or was held, responsible for misjudging me. He knows it as well as I do. So much to lose, lost so much already.

I nod.

'Yes, I was there and back in about five minutes. I went to the newsagent, the one just across the road from the school.'

'Nowhere else? You didn't go anywhere else?'

'No. Nowhere else, Mike.'

We sit in silence. I work hard to maintain eye contact. He breaks it first, leans forward, screws the top on the bottle of whisky, a signal it's over for now. The detail of people, the details I notice.

'It's late, Milly, you should go to bed. I need some time on my own.'

I turn round at the door just before I leave his study. One of his hands rests on the top of Phoebe's laptop, the other on the desk, fingers pointing, subconsciously maybe, in the direction of the phone.

'Mike, you need to give me my medication, and Saskia too. We need you.'

Up twenty-eight. Up another floor.
The banister on the right.

If I hadn't seen the text flash up on the screen of her phone, abandoned
next to the kettle during breakfast, Phoebe at the table.
Everything would have been different.
Everything.
'Come on, you sly beatch, what do you mean by D-day for
Dog-face tomorrow?' read the message.
Sender: Izzy
I left the scenery painting in the Great Hall to go and buy
snacks for everybody.
True.
The newsagent was the only place I went to.
False.
I ran all the way, five if you rush, less if you sprint.
I went up the stairs, up twenty-eight, up another floor, the banister
on the right. She was there. Screamed when she saw me.
Boo.
She went into her room, kicked the door shut behind her,
I followed. Get out, she said. Get away from me.
I took a step towards her. What are you doing, she asked.
Another step. She pushed past me, said, I'm calling Dad.
I didn't chase her, she would have run down the stairs,
I didn't want that. I walked out of her room. She was on the
landing, half sitting, half leaning on the banister.
Her safe place, from where she enjoyed tormenting her mother.
Fingerprints, hers, visible on the varnish. Fear as sweat, prickling her
pores. Overflowing. She was about to hit the call button.

337

Distracted.

Her, not me.

Another step towards her.

When somebody says it'll be the death of you. Believe them.

A second was all it took.

She was silent as she fell.

The Spanish tiles painted a new colour, her hair too.

*I ran all the way back, bearing goods for everyone from the
newsagent when I arrived.*

The officer's questions later on that night. Routine stuff really, he said.

No amount of training prepares them for the potential of children.

Oh Lord of the Flies.

I promised to be the best I could.

I promised to try.

Mike.

A kindly man.

I told him everything.

Well.

Almost everything.

Forgive me.

Acknowledgements

To the children and teenagers I looked after, it was a privilege. You were beyond brave, and without you, the basis of this book would not exist. To the staff I worked with over the years, for the laughter, when it so often could have been tears. Special mention to the team at the YPU in Edinburgh, my first job after qualifying. How we ever survived those night shifts is beyond me.

To my agent, Juliet Mushens, for scooping me up and making me real. For being the fastest reader I know with the most beautifully critical eye. You are a pocket rocket, a hustler and a lifelong friend. How lucky I am to know you.

Shout out to Sarah Manning – organizational dynamite – without your Post-it notes I would have been lost. And to Nathalie Hallam for taking over with ease. To #Team-Mushens as a whole, thank you for your support.

Jessica Leeke, my editor at Michael Joseph. Cheerleader, eagle-eye, anchor. You pushed me, yet held me. You gave me my brave. Ellie Hughes, my publicist, for knowing exactly what to do with me, and for being the chill to my hyper. Hattie Adam-Smith for being the divine, cool-as-a-cucumber, trilby-wearing, creative force behind all things marketing. Dream team all in. An extended thank you to the rest of the team at Michael Joseph and Penguin HQ. So many people doing so many things and with such warmth and enthusiasm. What a wonderful wing to be taken under by. Thank you all.

To Christine Kopprasch, my editor at Flatiron US, for believing, not just in this book, but in me as a writer. And an extended thank you, both to the rest of the team at Flatiron, and to Sasha Raskin, my US agent.

To Alex Clarke, who was involved in the acquisition of this book. Karen Whitlock for her sensitive and reassuring approach to copy-editing. To Richard Skinner for saying to me, 'Don't worry, Ali, just trust your instinct.' And I did, this book being the result.

To my family, with love.

And finally, the tribe! Peppered wonderfully around the world and without whom I'd never have had the courage to embark on this journey. You are too many, and there is too much, to thank you all individually for. So collectively, thank you for the colour, the creativity, the adventures, and the magic you bring into my life every day. And for loving me just the way I am, regardless. You completely brilliant, special dudes, I love you right back. Thank you thank you thank you, a million times over.